THE FIBROMYALGIA-TMJ CONNECTION

How Your Jaw, Teeth, Airway, and Meridians Affect Your Symptoms

Linda Faye Harris

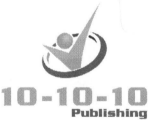

When my husband Steve was alive, he always encouraged me to write a book on fibromyalgia. When he passed away last year, I decided to follow his wishes, and so I dedicate this book to him.

Writing this book and interviewing and helping others has helped me deal with the grief of losing him, made me depend on the love and the guidance of the Lord, and filled my heart with joy in seeing the happiness in others as they improve their health.

Contents

TESTIMONIALS

Linda is my guardian angel. She assessed me after I had fibromyalgia for 36 years, and referred me to Dr Brock Rondeau DDS, who got me better. Linda saved my life.
Mary Catherine Aarssen, Wallaceburg, Ontario

I was a nursing student and had a car accident that changed my life. I suffered from headaches, could not sleep, developed TMJ, and felt like my whole life had crashed. I met Linda, and she interviewed me and guided me to the right dentists that could get me better. I am forever grateful.
Suzzane Rodgers, Wallaceburg, Ontario

I went to Linda's presentation on fibromyalgia, and she offered to interview me and do an assessment. She measured my upper palate which was narrow, that indicated my airway might be compromised. She guided me to Dr Felix Liao DDS, who identified by CAT scan that my airway and structure of my mouth was a problem. I cannot thank Linda enough for her passion to help me find the answer to my symptoms.
Brenda Smith, Petrolia, Ontario

Linda took one look at my granddaughter Mya and immediately knew that she did not sleep well, and had a high upper palate. She then asked if she had learning difficulties. She told me that Mya needs to have her mouth assessed for palate expansion by a dentist. She referred me to Dr Brock Rondeau DDS, who assessed Mya and suggested her tonsils were very large and needed to be removed. Then he fitted Mya with a palate expander. She is now sleeping better even though her treatment is not complete. Thank you, Linda, from the bottom of my heart.
Jill Nickles, Sarnia, Ontario

I have dentures and the dentist told me to take them out at night. Since I snored and did not sleep well and had difficulty finding my words when I talked, Linda suggested I leave my dentures in at night. I sleep better, do not snore as much, and have less difficulty finding my words. Thank you, Linda, for improving my life.
Pauline Chordash, Sombra, Ontario

As a nurse, Linda Harris has more training on TMJ, airway and head-jaw-neck alignment than nearly all doctors and dentists. Her extensive knowledge plus her TLC heart makes Linda Harris an angel among humans.
Dr Felix Liao DDS, Falls Church, Virginia

I am thankful to many people who influenced my journey of curiosity, and learning about the airways and the health impact on the overall body and mind. Proper jaw size, right bite and good sleep are critical to optimize our health and function at our best! Many chronic diseases are correlated with some airway constriction. Linda has an incredible level of knowledge about the jaw, airway, and meridians. Her passion to learn about dental malocclusion and how it affects the airways is incredible. Linda is very positive and always cares about others. The admiral task of writing this book is commendable!
Dr Stan D.D.S., London, Ontario

Linda Harris has created a must-read book for people who are, or know someone who is, suffering from chronic unresolved pain and dysfunction. She brings hope to those that were told to "live with your pain."
Dr Daniel R Gole D.D.S., Hastings, Michigan

ACKNOWLEDGEMENTS

So many people have walked with me on the road that led to these pages. The story written here would not be complete without any of you. I offer my deepest gratitude to the following people:

Steve, my late husband, who I was married to for 50 years. He has been the reason for my success in life. He always gave me positive reinforcement, and told me I was smart and capable of anything. He encouraged me to write this book to help others who suffered like me.

Kelly, my daughter, who not only supported me in my writing, but also was identified in one of my case studies.

Shawn, my son, who encourages me to continue my quest to help others to be symptom-free.

Judy and Bonnie, my university buddies who supported and encouraged me in my writing. Thank you for walking with me during the time of my symptoms and while I was researching my book. I am blessed with your friendship.

Judy and Jake, who helped me when my husband passed and called me daily. Thank you for believing in me and for your tireless encouragement.

My sister **Betty** and brother-in-law **Ernie**, my brother **Sam** and sister-in-law **Barbara**. I will be forever grateful for your love, and support during my dream of making this book possible.

All my **Cypress Lake buddies** who encourage me to be God's servant, and help others in His name.

Dr Brock Rondeau DDS and his staff: You are angels who not only got me better but helped many of the people that I interviewed, and treated their TMJ and airway problems.

Dr Dan Gole DDS: the head, neck and facial pain dentist who recognized that my bridge was on incorrectly I thank you from the bottom of my heart.

Dr Robert Dronyk: naturopathic chiropractor who gave me the dental meridian chart and was able to identify where my dental bridge was located without me opening my mouth since it coincided with the meridian dental chart.

Dr Stan DDS: who was very interested in me sharing my knowledge and research with her, as well as learning about the case studies of patients that I interviewed.

Dr Ralph Garcia DDS: TMJ dentist from Tampa. Thank you for sharing your expertise and case studies with me.

Dr Felix Liao DDS: Holistic Mouth Solution dentist. Thank you for educating me about the importance of the anatomy of the mouth and how it relates to our airway and overall health, and sharing your case studies.

Dr Dawn Ewing: Thank you for sharing your research on the organ/dental meridian, and confirming the use of the dental meridian chart when assessing patients.

Dr Lisa Sanders, although you don't know me, I thank you for looking for answers for patients that are difficult to diagnose. Your passion encourages me to search for the answers related to fibromyalgia.

Linda Harris

Lewis Howes, your *School of Greatness* podcast with your many guests gave me the encouragement to fulfil my dream of writing a book, and stay in the now after my husband passed.

I cannot thank **Diana Wisemen** enough for helping me with the illustrations in my book. Diana, you are a special friend!

FOREWORD

I first met Linda Harris in 1997, who was a registered nurse who came to my office suffering from fibromyalgia and temporomandibular joint dysfunction (TMD).

After going to Dr Gole DDS in Michigan to have her dental bridge removed, Linda came to me to have an intra-oral appliance to move her lower jaw forward. When you eliminate the click you eliminate 94% of the TMD symptoms. When I was able to relieve her migraines and painful symptoms, we became friends, and she referred many patients to my office over the past 25 years.

She has now decided to write this book on TMD (temporal mandibular joint dysfunction) and cranio-facial pain in order to help patients to understand the problem and learn that they can get treatment.

I gave Linda many of my dental books on TMD so that she could become more knowledgeable and help more patients. To assist her with her quest in TMD, I arranged for her to go to the US to attend the Head, Neck and Facial Pain TMJ Assistant Course. I have asked Linda to speak to my team about what she has learned about the jaw, airway, breathing problems, and meridians that affect patients.

According to the American Dental Association, TMD is prevalent in approximately 34% of the adult population. Children can also have TMD. The problem is very significant because the vast majority of dentists, medical doctors and specialists receive no training in this important disorder that affects so many patients.

Based on her years of experience and on the number of patients she has been able to help, Linda has written a very informative book to help patients understand how to help correct this painful and life-changing TMJ (temporal mandibular joint) disorder. Patients must seek out dentists who have been specially trained to treat these patients.

I am extremely proud of Linda, who has dedicated her life to helping patients eliminate TMD and achieve an improved level of health. Linda is a credit to the nursing profession, and has set an outstanding example of someone who has positively influenced the lives of hundreds of patients.

**Dr Brock Rondeau, D.D.S. I.B.O., D.A.B.C.P., D-A.C.S.D.D.,
D.A.B.D.S.M.,.A.B.C.D.S.M. Medicine TMJ Dentist, Orthodontics
and Sleep Apnea Dentist
London, Ontario**

Chapter 1

Discovering the Secret
Behind My Own Fibromyalgia

The meaning of life is to find your gift.
The purpose of life is to give it away.
~ Pablo Picasso

Who would ever think that your teeth and position of your jaw would have such a pivotal effect on your health? I am a nurse and my story may surprise you.

I believe that my journey began when I was a child: I was born the second of three children. Of the 3 of us, I was the only one who had a major accident when I was young. I had gone down a hill and had flown off my bike head first. Although I healed from my injuries I believe that there was damage done to my jaw that went undiscovered. Was the disc in my jaw displaced? Additionally I had an overbite, my bottom teeth were behind my upper teeth. I am not sure if this was a result of the accident or of my natural anatomy, but it would eventually become an important piece of the puzzle.

My jaw would click when I opened my mouth, but no one in the medical or dental fields seemed to think that this was a problem. When I was 15 years old, I started getting migraine headaches, and when I went to nursing school at age 17 my headaches occurred more often and became more debilitating.

When I got my migraine headaches the pain was usually over my left eye. It always seemed to be the left side of my head that was affected. I realized that this was also on the side that my jaw clicked. My headaches were often violently painful. I was frequently nauseated and often got some relief when I would vomit. The room would have to be dark and I could not tolerate any noise in the house. The blood vessels seem to pulsate in my head. Anyone who has had migraines can certainly relate.

During my 20's I was prescribed Cafergot suppositories for my migraine headaches. Eventually I was given Imitrex injections that I administered. I was also given intravenous Decadron, a strong steroid, at the hospital. This medication gave me rapid pain relief, but I only took this medication if I was at the hospital working when I got the headache, and was unable to drive home.

In my 30's , I was in a migraine research study in London Ontario where I was given medication and I did not know if I was taking a drug or a placebo. I had to be pulled from the study by my medical doctor. I found out that I was on Inderal, a beta blocker, which slowed down my heart rate, and made me so tired that I had difficulty functioning in my job.

I was a head nurse at a hospital in Canada, I had a tooth pulled and did not like the look of having a tooth missing. The dentist suggested placing a bridge on my upper left molars. This was done the day before Labour Day. Three days later, I became sensitive to smells i.e. perfume, or tobacco and would faint if the smell was strong. I fainted over ten times between September 7 and the middle of October 1995. The fainting stopped abruptly when my temporary bridge popped off. Two weeks later, on October 31 I had an appointment to have the permanent bridge placed.

It was after the permanent bridge was placed that I started fainting again. I had recently been promoted from head nurse to Director of In-patient Services at a small hospital in Wallaceburg, Ontario. The Administration assumed that my fainting was related to stress or anxiety in regards to my new job. I had to take time off work. I saw a cardiologist who ordered a holter monitor: the results showed that there were no abnormalities. I was also referred to a neurologist about my fainting. Two weeks later my fainting stopped after I returned to the dentist with a toothache under my bridge. An x-ray showed an abscess in the root of one of the teeth holding on my bridge. He drilled through my bridge and there was a foul smell. Due to the infection I asked if I should go on antibiotics, but my dentist told me that it was unnecessary since my tooth was draining. My dentist did not do root canals which I would need. I travelled to London, Ontario to see an endodontist to have the root canal done. This dentist had been talking to my family dentist and knew about my fainting, and that I thought it was related to my teeth. He thought it was related to my anxiety. That response made me sit up in the dental chair. I told him I did not want him looking after my teeth and walked out of his office.

Knowing that I had to get a root canal I went to see my sister-in-law who worked in neurology research at the University Hospital in London. I thought she would probably know a good endodontist. When I arrived I discovered that she would not return to her office for a few hours. While I waited I decided to go to the dental school library which was attached to the hospital. While looking for the library, I bumped into a young man, and asked him where the dental library was located. He asked what I wanted to know, as he was a fourth year dental student. I told him about the hole in my bridge and the abscessed tooth. He asked if I was on antibiotics. When I told him that I was not, he told me that I should be on them. He suggested that I go down to the dental school and tell them that he had sent me. I was prescribed antibiotics and told to come back in 3 days for a root canal to be done at the dental school.

During the root canal I thought someone had spilled bleach. The 4th year student working on me said there was no bleach spilled. He did mention that he had bleach on the cotton with which he was cleaning the root of my tooth. I had, according to him, very long roots which navigated to my sinuses. After the root canal was finished, I had no further problems with strong smells like perfume. Finally I thought, my dental problems were resolved. Unfortunately, that was not to be. Over the next six months, since the work on my teeth had started, I now had a cluster of new symptoms which appeared primarily on my left side, neck and chest. This was in addition to difficulty sleeping since the dental bridge was placed.

My symptoms included, but were not limited to:

- Shoulder and neck pain, unable to turn my head to the left
- Bruising
- Lack of concentration
- Came out with the wrong words when I spoke
- Twitching in my Left eye
- Blurred vision Left eye
- Black spots floating in front of my eyes
- Shoulder rolled forward
- Dreams
- Snoring
- Biting the Left side of my cheek
- Tongue scalloped around edges
- Difficulty swallowing pills
- Grinding my teeth
- Chills and sweating mostly at night
- Difficulty sleeping
- Panic attacks
- Soreness in my chest, rapid pulse
- Sciatica, low back pain
- Pain down left side, tendonitis, carpal tunnel
- Cold hands and feet
- Constipation, indigestion and bloating
- Several sore throats
- Balance was off, running into walls
- Left ankle seemed to twist easily
- Catch my L big toes when I walked
- Extreme fatigue

Several months later, I went to my doctor, who diagnosed me with fibromyalgia and put me on a low dose of amitriptyline at bedtime, and Ibuprofen for generalized pain during the day. In 1996, the doctor knew very little about fibromyalgia, and this was standard treatment at the time.

I did not go back to working at the hospital, because I was unable to sleep. My entire life was turned upside down. Eight months later I started fainting again. The medical profession seemed to have done all it could at the moment, so I thought that going to the dentist first might be of benefit. The tooth was x-rayed and I had another abscess tooth underneath the root canal that had previously been done. The fainting stopped after I had another root canal completed on the same tooth. While the dental work resolved the fainting, other symptoms were still developing. Although I was no longer working in the hospital, I was a CPR instructor. While taking my recertification course, two people taking the course with me mentioned that I had been asleep for at least ten minutes twice during a two hour period. I didn't even realize it. Had I now developed narcolepsy?

I made an appointment with a naturopathic chiropractor, Dr. Dronyk regarding my fibromyalgia symptoms. I told him that I believed that my symptoms had all started with my dental work. Without looking in my mouth he told me where my bridge was located. He told me that he had used a dental-meridian chart similar to the one shown on the next page. He used it to determine where my bridge was located.

Organs	Joints	Vertebrae	Endocrine	Systems	Sensory	Muscles	Sinus	Patient's Right Side
Heart Terminal Ileum Ileo-Cecal Area	Ulnar side of shoulder, Hand and Elbow Plantar side of Foot Toes Sacro-Iliac	C - 1, 2, 7 TH - 1, 5, 6, 7 S - 1, 2		Peripheral Nerves Energy Exchange	Middle Ext. Ear Tongue	Psoas		32
Lung, Large Intestine Ileo-Cecal Area	Radial side of Shoulder, Hand and Elbow Foot Big Toe	C - 1, 2, 5, 6, 7 TH - 2, 3, 4 L - 4, 5		Arteries (31) Veins (30)	Nose	Quadriceps (31) Gracilis (30) Sartorius (30)	Ethmoid	31 30
Esophagus Stomach Pancreas Pylorus Pyloric Antrum	Anterior Hip Anterior Knee Medial Ankle Jaw	C - 1, 2 TH - 11, 12 L - 1	Ovary and Testicle (28)	Lymph (29) Breast	Tongue	Pect Maj Sternal (29) Quadratus Lumborum (28) Hamstring	Maxillary	29 28
Liver Gallbladder Biliary Ducts	Posterior Knee Hip Lateral Ankle	C - 1, 2 TH - 8, 9, 10	Ovary Testicle		Anterior Eye	Gluteus Maximus	Sphenoid	27
Kidney Bladder Ovary/Testicle Prostate/Uterus Rectum/Anus	Posterior Knee Sacro-coccygeal Posterior ankle	C - 1, 2 L - 2, 3 S - 3, 4, 5 Coccyx	Adrenals			Tensor Fasciae Latae (26) Pyriformis (26) Gluteus Medius (25)	Frontal Sphenoid	26 25
Kidney Bladder Ovary/Testicle Prostate/Uterus Rectum/Anus	Posterior Knee Sacro-coccygeal Posterior ankle	C - 1, 2 L - 2, 3 S - 3, 4, 5 Coccyx	Adrenals			Tensor Fasciae Latae (23) Pyriformis (23) Gluteus Medius (24)	Frontal Sphenoid	24 23
Liver Biliary Ducts	Posterior Knee Hip Lateral Ankle	C - 1, 2 TH - 8, 9, 10	Ovary Testicle		Anterior Eye	Gluteus Maximus	Sphenoid	22
Esophagus Stomach Spleen	Anterior Hip Anterior Knee Medial Ankle Jaw	C - 1, 2 TH - 11, 12 L - 1	Ovary and Testicle (21)	Lymph (20) Breast	Tongue	Pect Maj Sternal (20) Quadratus Lumborum (21) Hamstring	Maxillary	21 20
Lung Large Intestine	Radial side of Shoulder, Hand and Elbow Foot Big Toe	C - 1, 2, 5, 6, 7 TH - 2, 3, 4 L - 4, 5		Arteries (18) Veins (19)	Nose	Quadriceps (18) Gracilis (19) Sartorius (19)	Ethmoid	19 18
Heart Ileum Jejunum	Ulnar side of shoulder, Hand and Elbow, Plantar side of Foot, Toes, Sacro-Iliac	C - 1, 2, 7 TH - 1, 5, 6, 7 S - 1, 2		Peripheral Nerves Energy Exchange	Middle Ext. Ear Tongue	Psoas		17

Dental Meridian Chart Copyright 2002 Courtesy of Dr. Dawn Ewing Holistic Alternatives www.drdawn.net

MERIDIAN TOOTH CHART - Description available on pages 82-92.

Patient's Right Side	Sinus	Muscles	Sensory	Systems	Endocrine	Vertebrae	Joints	Organs
1		Trapezius	Internal Ear Tongue	Central Nervous Limbic	Ant. Pituitary	C - 1, 2, 7 TH - 1, 5, 6, 7 S - 1, 2	Ulnar side of Shoulder, Hand and Elbow Plantar side of Foot, Toes, Sacro-Iliac	Heart Terminal Ileum Duodenum
2 3	Maxillary	Abdominal (2) Latissimus (3)	Oropharynx Larynx Tongue	Breast	Thyroid (3) Parathyroid (2)	C - 1, 2 TH - 11, 12 L - 1	Jaw, Ant. Hip Ant. Knee Medial Ankle	Pancreas Stomach Esophagus
4 5	Ethmoid	Diaphragm (4) Pectoralis Maj. Clavicular Coracobrachialis Popliteus (5)	Nose	Breast (4)	Thymus (4) Post. Pituitary (5)	C - 1, 2, 5, 6, 7 TH - 2, 3, 4 L - 4, 5	Radial side of Shoulder, Hand and Elbow Foot Big Toe	Lung Large Intestine Bronchi
6	Sphenoid	Deltoid Ant. Serratus	Posterior Eye		Intermediate Pituitary Hypothalamus	C - 1, 2 TH - 8, 9, 10	Posterior Knee Hip Lateral Ankle	Liver Gallbladder Biliary Ducts
7 8	Frontal Sphenoid	Subscapularis (7) Neck-Flex and Ext (8)	Nose		Pineal	C - 1, 2 L - 2, 3 S - 3, 4, 5 Coccyx	Posterior Knee Sacro-coccygeal Posterior Ankle	Kidney, Bladder Ovary/Testicle Prostate/Uterus Rectum/Anus
9 10	Frontal Sphenoid	Subscapularis(10) Neck-Flex and Ext (9)	Nose		Pineal	C - 1, 2 L - 2, 3 S - 3, 4, 5 Coccyx	Posterior Knee Sacro-coccygeal Posterior Ankle	Kidney, Bladder Ovary/Testicle Prostate/Uterus Rectum/Anus
11	Sphenoid	Deltoid Ant. Serratus	Posterior Eye		Intermediate Pituitary Hypothalamus	C - 1, 2 TH - 8, 9, 10	Posterior Knee Hip Lateral Ankle	Liver Biliary Ducts
12 13	Ethmoid	Diaphragm (13) Pectoralis Maj. Clavicular Coracobrachialis Popliteus (12)	Nose	Breast (13)	Thymus (13) Post. Pituitary (12)	C - 1, 2, 5, 6, 7 TH - 2, 3, 4 L - 4, 5	Radial side of Shoulder, Hand and Elbow Foot Big Toe	Lung Large Intestine Bronchi
14 15	Maxillary	Abdomial (15) Lattisimus (14)	Oropharynx Larynx Tongue	Breast	Thyroid (14) Parathyroid (15)	C - 1, 2 TH - 11, 12 L - 1	Jaw, Ant. Hip Ant. Knee Medial Ankle	Spleen Stomach Esophagus
16		Trapezius	Internal Ear Tongue	Central Nervous Limbic	Ant. Pituitary	C - 1, 2, 7 TH - 1, 5, 6, 7 S - 1, 2	Ulnar side of shoulder, Hand and Elbow, Plantar side of Foot, Toes, Sacro-Iliac	Heart Duodenum Jejunum Ileum

Dental Meridian Chart Copyright 2002 Courtesy of Dr. Dawn Ewing Holistic Alternatives www.drdawn.net

MERIDIAN TOOTH CHART - Description available on pages 82-92.

7

Tooth # 13 is the one that pertained to me. I had the symptoms down the Meridian of the tooth that was connected to my dental bridge. The correspondences and my symptoms were so closely tied:

Dental Chart Tooth # 13
- Ethmoid cells. (Lining of the sinus) - I had problem with smells and my sinuses
- Shoulder, elbow I had tendonitis
- Hand radial, I had carpal tunnel
- Foot, my left ankle twisted easily
- Big toe I would catch my big toe when I walked
- C 5,6,7 cervical spine - I could not turn my head all the way to my left
- T 2,3,4, mid chest I had soreness in my chest
- L4,5 sciatic nerve pain that radiates from lower back down my left leg
- Lung left I did not notice problems with my lungs
- Large intestines - I was constipated
- Thymus - It is an immune system organ located behind the breast bone
- Breast - I had thickening in my breast requiring mammogram

Dr Dronyk, the naturopathic chiropractor, concluded that my physical symptoms were definitely related to my teeth. I thought, hoped, that finally I would get some help. I made an appointment with a new dentist in Sarnia. I showed him the dental-meridian chart that I had received from Dr. Dronyk, which he had never seen before. Even with the chart and my history, he told me that the problem was not my teeth. I made an appointment with another dentist, I was once again told that I had no dental problems. He was adamant that no chiropractor was going to tell him that the root of the symptoms were dental in nature. After these consultations I realized that these dentists could not recognize my dental problem, since they only looked at me with my mouth open. If they had examined my bite, they would have quickly recognized that I was perhaps suffering from a crossbite and Temporomandibular Joint Dysfunction or TMJD. I was sure that my problem was still rooted in my teeth. I didn't feel that I had anywhere to turn any more. I had to try and make my way regardless of my medical issues. Six months after all the consultations, and so many disappointments, I signed up to go on a medical mission in Ecuador with Medical Missionary International.

On my flight to Ecuador I had to change planes in Miami. Although I had been lucky enough to get an aisle seat, a couple got on late, just prior to take off. The husband was sitting next to me and his wife was in a middle seat several rows ahead. I said that I would be willing to trade places with his wife so they could sit together. After switching seats, I began speaking to a lady from Kalamazoo Michigan. As it turned out, we both had daughters who played soccer. She told me that they just about lost their star soccer player. She had been experiencing pain in her arm and leg. She told me that one of her daughter's teammate's father was a "Head, Neck and Facial Pain Dentist" She said that he had worked on the star soccer player's teeth, and had managed to alleviate her symptoms. During the conversation, I mentioned that I had been dealing with issues with my teeth. I experienced pain in my arm and leg that coincided with getting my dental bridge. I truly believe that it was Divine intervention that led me to change my seat. I had been praying for relief. I believe that I was meant to speak with this person. I had never heard of a Head, Neck and Facial Pain dentist. The lady from Kalamazoo said she would write me a letter with Dr. Dan Gole's contact information.

The letter had arrived at my house when I returned from my medical mission in Ecuador. I called Dr. Gole and made an appointment. When I saw him the first time he handed me a mirror and asked if I thought my bite looked correct. I had a cross bite: my top and bottom teeth did not line up correctly. He also noted that my tongue was scalloped on the edges, and that it could not lay flat causing it to block my airway. He said my dental bridge had to come off. I agreed. After he removed the bridge and examined me, he indicated that the teeth that were pegged to hold onto the bridge were angled in such a way as to cause the bridge to sit too close to my cheek.

When he removed my dental bridge. It was AMAZING! My whole body relaxed: I could once again turn my head to the left; I stopped biting my cheek; I no longer fell asleep during the day. All of my fibromyalgia symptoms except my migraine headaches had DISAPPEARED. Dr. Gole knew he could help with fibromyalgia and had case studies summarized in his newsletter.

Finally, a dentist had listened to me, and his treatment had made me better. There is no way I would have found a dentist in Hastings, Michigan, so far away from my home in Canada. I truly believe that this was Divine intervention. I thanked God over and over again on my 3 hour drive home from Hastings, Michigan to Sombra, Ontario. I was virtually symptom free.

When I arrived home, my husband was thrilled that I was feeling better. He did, however, comment that my eyes look different. He said that he could now see more of the blue in my eyes. Although I had realized that my pupils were so much bigger for the last 2 years, I had attributed it to stress. As a nurse, I realized that my dental work and pain had caused me to be in fight and flight pattern over the last two years, causing my pupils to dilate. Dr. Gole told me, during my appointment, that my structural and dental stress had contributed to my stress level.

On the next page is Dr Gole's Stress Diagram. The first column is stress that can stay under the threshold of disease. The second column is someone who is close to the threshold of disease like me. Dental stress which is 24 hours a day and magnifies all other stressors. This is a dentist stress chart. Medical doctors only look at stress as being mental or psychological stress. Dr. Gole (dentist) said my dental bridge which was on incorrectly was causing me a great deal of dental and structural stress. After the dental bridge came off my whole body relaxed, as I said previously my pupils which were dilated returned to a normal size. My stress level had finally decreased.

Another change after my dental bridge was removed was the change in my mammogram. I had been having a mammogram every six months, times 2 due to thickening in my left breast. When I had my next six month mammogram they told me that the thickening was gone. When I got home from having the mammogram I took out my nursing anatomy book and looked at the lymphatic system.

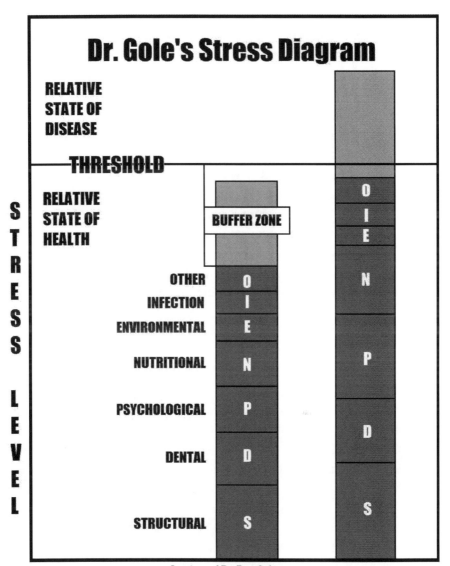

Courtesy of Dr. Dan Gole

I believe that since the muscles in my left chest were now relaxed once my dental bridge had been removed that the lymphatic system was now able to drain. The radiologist cancelled my next six month breast scan after discussing the changes with my doctor.

As treatments progressed, Dr Gole told me that my bottom jaw would need to come forward. He told me that I had an overbite, my bottom teeth were behind my top teeth. He told me that if my lower jaw was brought forward, it would bring my tongue forward as well. The changes in my anatomy would allow my airway to be more open. He further indicated that when my jaw came forward it would help my migraines. According to him, part of the reason for the migraines was that the blood vessels were being compressed in my jaw. Travelling was complicated by several snow storms that winter so I looked for a dentist in Canada that belongs to the Head, Neck and Facial Pain Dental Association. Now that I knew what to look for, I was lucky to find one about eighty miles away.

Dr. Brock Rondeau, the Canadian Head, Neck and Facial Pain dentist, fitted me with a double splint that I wore 24/7. Within six months, my bottom jaw had come forward 7mm. For the next part of my treatment, I was fitted with braces and he had erupted my back teeth by attaching elastics to my braces. I had braces for a year and a half, and then was fitted for a night splint to prevent my jaw from falling back when I was sleeping. During, and after all these treatments, my migraine headaches, the itching and pulsating in my ear, the sensitivity to light, and noise were finally gone. The blood vessels were no longer trapped behind the condyle of my jaw.

I had been a Head Nurse for 13 years and did not know that getting rid of my headaches was possible. I had been seeking help from a medical doctor. I then discovered that there were other options. For me, a TMJ dentist, is where I found my solution.

Dr Brock Rondeau, my Canadian TMJ (temporal mandibular joint) dentist, teaches dentists and orthodontics all over the United States, Canada and

Europe. During one of these teaching conferences in Toronto, ON, Canada, he had me come to his dental conference and relate my experience to the 200 attending dentists. I had also started to interview people with fibromyalgia. I completed the TMJ questionnaire and used the MERIDIAN chart that was given to me by Dr Dronyk, the naturopathic chiropractor, to identify which tooth was hitting first and the symptoms that the person was experiencing. I kept finding correspondence between the tooth issues and symptoms.

Mary Catherine Aarssen was the first lady that I interviewed. One of my nursing friends told me she had fibromyalgia and had been sick for many years. I contacted Mary Catherine and told her I had information about fibromyalgia that might be able to help her. When I arrived at her door, she started to cry and I asked her what was wrong. She told me that she had been to church that morning and asked God to take her life or send her an angel to get her better: I arrived at her door. I completed the Temporomandibular Joint (TMJ) questionnaire which indicated that she may have a TMJ dysfunction of her jaw. Mary did not have a bridge, as had been the root of my issue but she did have a malocclusion (bad bite) from missing teeth. She had been seeing the same dentist that had put my bridge in originally. He had made her a partial denture plate. It did not fit properly, so she had chosen not to wear it. This caused one tooth to hit in an uncomfortable way. We discovered that she had symptoms down the **meridian** of the tooth that hit first. Mary Catherine went to Dr Brock Rondeau (TMJ dentist), and got relief. She was so grateful for the results of the treatment, that she wrote him a letter. On the next page is a copy of the letter that she also wrote to the London Free Press about Dr Rondeau ten years after she was treated.

London Free Press July, 2008

Patient remembers dentist's efforts 10 years later

Words are never expressed enough for the people who do good in this world.

Ten years ago this month, I went to Dr. Brock Rondeau, a dentist in London. I was in terrible pain.

I had been in pain since 1967 and was diagnosed with chronic fatigue syndrome and fibromyalgia. I was bedridden for six months and couldn't walk or sit. Every day, I used to pray to die.

Dr. Rondeau and his staff listened to my cry for help. They carefully X-rayed and measured my jaw and I wore a daytime and nighttime splint. After persevering for 4½ years, I was all out of pain.

I am pain free today and I can't thank him and his staff enough for listening to me.

Mary Catherine Aarssen

Port Lambton

It was at this point that I realized that there was something potentially as life altering for others as it had been for me. In order to get the word out and help other people with fibromyalgia, I spoke at ladies groups, the library and anywhere I could, in an effort to help other people. I truly believed that God led me to the path of healing, so I could help others. I spoke at the library in London, and was approached by a dentist and a chiropractor who were in the audience. The chiropractor said that I was right on target, with what I was presenting about the Fibromyalgia-TMJ Connection. I know that several people were very positively impacted by my presentations.

One lady, Mrs. Babcock, whom I had met at one of the ladies church groups meetings, suffered from ringing in her ears. She made an appointment with Dr Rondeau. Her medical doctor told her that a dentist could not help ringing in the ear, and discouraged her from seeing him. Dr. Rondeau made her a splint and she had dental work done. The ringing in her ears went away. After discovering that his patient had gotten relief, the medical doctor asked for the name of the dentist, as he also had ringing in his ears.

As I expanded my speaking engagements, I began to speak at dental conferences. Many of the dentists that I met at Dr Rondeau's dental conference had their patients call me. I would interview them over the phone: I did the TMJ questionnaire and asked them which tooth hit first and I would follow the meridian line down on the dental chart of the tooth that hit first. I started to see convergences. I interviewed six women with Sjogren's Syndrome: all six were hitting their front teeth first. They had dry eyes, dry mouth, dry cough, and fatigue symptoms down the front teeth meridian. (Refer to the meridian chart, page 6&7.)

I later attended a conference in London, Ontario hosted by Dr Hall, a medical doctor from California, on Fibromyalgia. He discussed typical fibromyalgia presentations in patients and highlighted the lack of sleep that often shows up in these patients. Many patients end up developing autoimmune diseases, and if one does not sleep well, one has a tendency to gain weight.

At the end of the conference I lined up to talk to Dr Hall about fibromyalgia. I was the third in line, and the lady talking to Dr Hall in front of me was mentioning that her sixteen-year-old daughter had fibromyalgia and had been in bed most of the last six months. It was then the next lady in line to talk to Dr Hall. The lady with the sixteen-year-old daughter with fibromyalgia walked by me. I asked her if her daughter had anything wrong with her teeth before she got fibromyalgia. Her eyes got big as saucers, and she affirmed that her daughter had flown off her bike and knocked her two front teeth out. She said that they saved the teeth roots and I that the dentist had wired them back in place. To me, this just reinforced the hypothesis that fibromyalgia may have a dental connection.

As I continued my journey, I was increasingly convinced that there was a link between jaw/dental issues and Fibromyalgia. I explored this link more when I went to a class reunion with two of my girlfriends. I told them to look for classmates that had a narrow smile; a smile where you could just see at most six front teeth when they smiled. These people usually had a high upper palate and did not sleep well. We noticed that there were two classmates that had narrow smiles and high palates and both had teeth pulled when they had braces when they were young. After speaking with them, I discovered that both of them did not sleep well and had autoimmune diseases. This confirmed, for me, the observations that Dr Hall had mentioned in his lecture. Did the removal of their teeth when they were young cause a narrow upper palate? I continued exploring those links.

Now that I was feeling better I went back to work. I live on the Canadian-American border and took a night job at the State Prison. I realized that this was meant to be. This medical situation is one of the few places where a person's dental and medical charts are kept together. I continued to research the link in a more comprehensive way. When I took my break at night, I would look at the dental records of inmates that had TMJD. (temporomandibular jaw dysfunction) When I read their medical records, I was able to identify many similarities in their symptoms. While I worked at the prison I shared my dental research with a co-worker. This officer's son had ADD (attention deficit

16

disorder) symptoms, did not sleep well and had a narrow upper palate. His family took him to Dr, Gole, the TMJ dentist in the USA that had first diagnosed me. The doctor expanded the boy's upper palate and the child started to sleep better and his behaviour totally changed. He calmed down and did much better in school. In another situation, another officer's mother broke her dentures. The loss of her dentures coincided with her having balance problems, she had to use a cane. After Dr Gole replaced the dentures, her bite was balanced, and she was then able to walk independently once again. Eventually, I switched jobs and started working full time at a hospital in Mt Clemens, Michigan, and I had very little time to continue my dental research. It was not until I retired 20 years later from my job at Select Specialty Hospital that my husband encouraged me to write a book on The Fibromyalgia -TMJ Connection.

I took a book writing course, and here I am putting my words to paper.

Chapter 2

What is Fibromyalgia?

It is health that is real wealth, not pieces of gold and silver.
~ Mahatma Gandhi

What is Fibromyalgia Syndrome FMS?

Fibromyalgia syndrome (FMS) is a combination of the Latin root "fibro" (connective tissue fibres), "my" (muscle),"al" (pain, and "gia" (condition of). The word syndrome simply means a group of signs and symptoms that occur together which characterizes a particular abnormality.

According to Wikipedia, fibromyalgia (FMS) is a medical condition of unknown etiology (cause) characterized by chronic widespread pain and a heightened pain response to pressure. Other symptoms include tiredness to a degree that normal activities are affected, sleep problems, and cognitive dysfunction. Some people also report restless leg syndrome, bowel and bladder problems, numbness and tingling and sensitivity to noise, light or temperature. Individuals with FMS also often have Raynaud's Syndrome, which is characterized by a decreased blood flow in fingers, toes, and other extremities, caused by spasms in the blood vessels in those areas. The spasms are often a result of cold, stress, or emotional distress.

With FMS, the standard medical tests usually come back negative. Doctors often become very frustrated and question if the problem is psychological. There are no laboratory tests to diagnose fibromyalgia. When doctors are unable to diagnose the problem, they will frequently refer the client to a specialist i.e. rheumatologist. Although there may be several underlying causes for FMS, what if the main cause is not a medical problem but a dental problem? If that was true, then a general physician or other medical doctors will never find a solution.

In 1990, the diagnostic tender points for FMS was defined by the American College of Rheumatology:

"The presence of unexplained widespread pain or aching, persistent fatigue, generalized morning stiffness, non-refreshing sleep, and multiple tender points. Most patients with these symptoms must have at least 11 of the 18 specific tender points to be diagnosed with FMS."

Fibromyalgia Trigger Point Sites

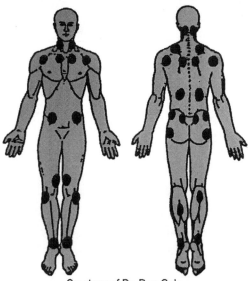

Courtesy of Dr. Dan Gole

20

There is some suggestion that FMS may be inherited, according to research. This means that approximately half of the children of FMS parents have the potential to eventually develop FMS on an autosomal dominant basis. TMJ dentists suggest that the reason for this may be the similarity in the jaw structure, overbite, or a narrow upper palate. This may play a role in the inherited tendency to develop FMS.

There are no lab tests to diagnose fibromyalgia since because there are so many symptoms that overlap other conditions, your doctor may choose to <u>rule out these</u> other conditions that have similar symptoms. Blood tests may include:

- Complete blood count
- Erythrocyte sedimentation rate
- Cyclic citrullinated peptide test
- Rheumatoid factor
- Thyroid function tests
- Antinuclear antibodies
- Celiac serology
- Vitamin D

If there is a chance that you may be suffering from sleep apnea, your doctor may also recommend an overnight sleep study.

According to medical doctors there is no cure for this disorder, and patients are told that they must learn to manage their symptoms or take heavy medications. There may, however, be another option. Exploring your symptoms with a knowledgeable TMJ dentist may allow you to discover some solutions that medical doctors are not able to address because their focus is not the jaw, airway, teeth or meridians.

According to the Mayo Clinic's website, in the past, doctors would check 18 specific points on a person's body to see how many of them were painful when pressed firmly. Newer guidelines from the American College of Rheumatology don't require a tender point exam. Instead, the main factor needed for fibromyalgia diagnosis is widespread pain throughout the body for at least three months. To meet the criteria, you must have pain in at least four of these five following areas:

- **Left upper region**: including shoulder, arm and jaw
- **Right upper region**: including shoulder, arm and jaw
- **Left lower region**: including hip, buttocks or leg
- **Right lower region**: including hip buttock or leg
- **Axial region**: which includes neck, back, chest or abdomen

Dr Devin Starlanyl in her book <u>Fibromyalgia and Chronic Myofascial Pain Syndrome</u> identifies several symptoms of fibromyalgia. Included in her very comprehensive list are:

- Growing pains as a child
- Attract mosquitoes and black flies
- Fatigue
- Mottled or blotchy skin
- Double jointed
- Crave carbohydrates
- Frequent yeast infection
- Overgrowing connective tissue, nail ridges
- Wide body aches and pains
- Have sleep apnea
- Generalized itching
- Experience frequent frustration
- Experience unusual reactions to medication
- Thick mucus secretions
- Inability to sweat or extreme night morning sweats
- Have patches of skin with painful network of fine veins and capillaries
- Extreme susceptibility to infection
- Delayed reaction until the next day if too active physically
- Get the shakes when you are hungry

- Bruise easily
- Recent weight change loss or gain
- Noise of fluorescent light bother you
- Have electromagnetic sensitivity-affected by electrical storms and when there is a full moon
- Experience numbness or tingling
- Does writing with a fingernail on your skin leave a red welt
- Have had a serious illness, surgeries or physical trauma

Symptoms of Fibromyalgia Generally Associated with Trigger Points in the Head (Myofascial Pain):

- Motor Coordination problems
- Unusual degree of clumsiness
- Sinus stuffiness
- Frequent runny nose
- Trouble swallowing
- Ear pain
- Fluctuating blood pressure
- Dry eyes, nose and mouth
- Problems swallowing and chewing
- Prickling "electric face"
- Red or tearing eyes
- Popping or clicking of the jaw
- Itchy ear
- Grind and clench your teeth
- Unexplained toothache
- Eye pain
- Sensitive to light
- Night driving problems
- Double vision, blurry vision, or changing vision
- Dark specks that float in your vision
- Words jump of the page or disappear when you stare at them
- Frequent headaches

- Migraines
- Stiff neck
- Dizziness when you turn your head
- Sore spot on top of the head

Symptoms of Fibromyalgia Caused by Tender Points in the Shoulder, Back, Arm, Chest, Buttocks and Groin:

- Pain mid-shoulder when you carry a purser wear heavy clothes
- Pain when you write, a changing signature, and /or illegible handwriting
- Extremities turn colour or blanche with the cold (often referred to as Raynaud's Syndrome)
- Esophageal reflux
- Shortness of breath
- Hypersensitive nipples or breast pain
- Frozen Shoulder
- Painful weak grasp that sometimes lets go
- Chest tightness
- Hiatal hernia
- Mitral valve prolapse
- Intestinal cramps, bloating
- Nausea
- Irritable bladder and/or bowel
- Burning or foul smelling urine
- Pain with intercourse
- Menstrual problems such as severe cramping, delayed irregular periods, with a great deal of bleeding
- Impotence
- Low back pain, sciatica

Symptoms of Fibromyalgia Caused by Leg, and Foot Trigger Points:

- Shin splints
- Stumble over your own feet

- Upper/lower leg cramps
- Muscle cramps and twitches everywhere
- Buckling knees
- Foot pain
- Tight hamstrings
- Numbness hypersensitivity (ants crawling under skin, on the outer thighs; burning and redness on the inner thigh)
- Restless leg syndrome
- Staggering walk and balance problem
- First walk in a.m. feels like walking nails common in flat foot, or high arches
- Weak ankles

A highly recommended resource to expand your knowledge of FMS is Dr Devin Starlanyl's book **Fibromyalgia & Chronic Myofascial Pain Syndrome A Survival Manual** as she explains the interrelationship between trigger points and provides a more comprehensive list of fibromyalgia symptoms.

If you have been diagnosed with fibromyalgia, or if you think you have, I suggest you make a list of those symptoms. There is another possibility with respect to the root of these symptoms that we will be exploring in the chapter on meridians.

Trigger Points

The term trigger point was coined in 1942 by Dr. Janet Travell to describe clinical findings in her book Myofascial Pain and Dysfunction The Trigger Point Manual.

1. Pain related to discrete irritable points in skeletal muscle or fascia, not caused by acute local trauma inflammation, degeneration, neoplasm or infection.

2. The pain from trigger points can be felt as a nodule or band in the muscle and a twitch response can be listed on stimulation of the trigger point.

3. Palpitation of the trigger-points reproduces the patient complaining of pain, with the pain radiating in a distribution of the muscle and/or nerve. Patients can have a trigger point in their upper trapezius muscle and once compressed feel pain in their forearm hand and fingers. ie. A patient who is having heart pain can feel pain in the arm or jaw.

According to Dr Janet Travell (medical doctor) trigger points form only in muscles. There is a local contraction in the small number of muscle fibers in a large muscle or muscle bundle. This, in turn, can **pull on tendons and ligaments** associated with muscle and can **cause pain within a joint** where there are no muscles. This is why when one has pain in one's joints x-rays, MRI and CAT Scans are negative.

Most tension headaches are caused by trigger points. These knots or mini-spasms cause pain to travel in predictable patterns to different areas of the body, often nowhere near the tight area.

In the picture below the X marks the trigger point. The shaded area shows the pain pattern related to the trigger point.

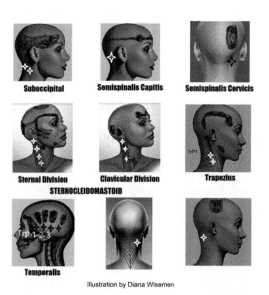

Illustration by Diana Wisemen

The pictures on page 26 are related to the trigger points in the neck and head.

Simons, D. G., Simons, L. S., & Travell, J. G. (1999). Travell & Simons Myofascial Pain and Dysfunction: The Trigger Point Manual. Baltimore: Williams & Wilkins Myofascial Pain and Dysfunction. The Trigger Point Manual Volume 1. Upper Half of Body Second Edition. David G Simon, MD, Janet Travell,MD, Lois S. Simons, P.T. 1999

Symptoms of Fibromyalgia Associated with Trigger Points in the Muscles of the Head (Myofascial Pain):

- Headaches
- Ringing in the ear
- Dizziness
- Migraines
- Stiff neck
- Sore spot on top on the head
- Vision problems
- Spots in front of the eyes
- Unexplained toothache
- Grind and clench teeth
- Itchy ears
- Problem with swallowing and chewing
- Dry eyes
- Dry mouth
- Chronic dry cough
- Ear pain
- Sinus stuffiness
- Unusual degree of clumsiness and motor coordination problems.

These are Myofascial Pain Symptoms. Each one of the above symptoms in the body are explained in further detail in Dr Devin Starlanyl book Fibromyalgia & Chronic Myofascial Pain Syndrome. (Devin Starlanyl, M.D. Mary Ellen Copeland M.S., M.A 1996

According to Dr Brock Rondeau, a TMJ dentist, in his course manual: <u>Diagnosis and Treatment of TMD (temporal mandibular dysfunction)</u> Dec 17, 2020, " one of the main causes of trigger points is actually temporomandibular joint (TMJ) problems due to the lack of proper posterior vertical dimension, which results in the tip of the lower jaw bone (mandible) being displaced posteriorly causing impingement of the nerves and blood vessel (superior carotid artery) in that area. This reduction in blood supply to the muscles that open and close the lower jaw (mandible) ,can lead to the muscles going into spasm with resultant discomfort."

If the muscles that open and close the jaw (mandible) become shortened, this can lead to bruxism and grinding. Patients will brux as a way of preventing their muscles from going into spasm. The dentist must palpate the muscles around the TMJ carefully to check for trigger points. If there are several trigger points in this area of the muscle contraction, the dentist knows that there is a problem with proper jaw and teeth position.

Some people have decreased vertical dimension in their mouth if they are missing teeth, if their back teeth have not erupted all the way, their teeth are worn down, or the disc in the jaw has been displaced due to a whiplash or accident. Any or all of these things can cause TMJ dysfunction. Decreased vertical dimension can cause muscle spasm and cause a cascade of trigger points and symptoms. Consulting a good TMJ or Airway dentist will allow you to assess if your pain or symptoms in your head and neck are related to a high crown, teeth missing, or the position of the jaw.

Trigger points in your neck can cause symptoms in your arms and fingers and back. The trigger points, in the rest of your body, can also be triggered by your jaw, teeth, and meridians. The trigger points in the trunk and legs will be explained when you take the meridians into consideration in a later chapter.

Linda Harris

Dental Solution to Fibromyalgia

This article was in Dr. Gole's "ToothPrints" (Teeth do more than just chew) newsletter. He relates the following in a case study:

Fibromyalgia (from Dr Gole's case studies)

Patient is a 35-year-old female patient suffering for five years with the following symptoms: achy, stiff, painful muscles throughout the body, headaches, fatigue, disturb sleep, inability to concentrate, depression, food allergies, bruised easily, irritable bowel syndrome, hands are constantly white and cold, irritable, and weak muscles making exercise excruciating.

The cause of these symptoms is not clear but they mysteriously appeared after her last pregnancy. She was eventually diagnosed with fibromyalgia. The stiffness and pain deep within the muscle makes even simple tasks seem difficult. Emotional tension, hormonal swings aggravated the knotting in the muscles. "Pills and learning to live with it "were the suggested conservative options along with exercise and physical treatment.

Treatment: The resultant force vector technique RVF Analysis (muscle testing) revealed tender muscles throughout the body. Functional testing showed a positive link to the teeth, indicating that favourable changes could be made through a dental perspective.

Phase 1 Treatment consisting of an oral orthotic appliance (splint), and physical medicine modalities eliminated 85 to 90% of the patient symptoms in eight weeks.(the splint prevents the teeth from touching)

Phase 2 Treatment using RVF technique (muscle testing), put the patient back in her own teeth in four weeks. Fine-tuning the bite has made life enjoyable again.

29

A six month post-treatment evaluation showed a 95-98% reduction in symptoms with a return to normal life-style for a mother with two children.

MEDICAL DOCTORS SOLUTION TO FIBROMYALGIA

According to Dr Benjamin Abraham, a pain management specialist from the Cleveland Clinic, fibromyalgia is a disorder of pain processing. He explains how treatment involves a team of specialists and engages both the mind and the body. When one is treated for fibromyalgia at the Cleveland Clinic they structure a one hour appointment with a Neurologist and explain the newest research. After that one hour, they spend another hour with these patients, coordinating a Pain Psychologist, someone that specializes in these psychological treatment methods. The two hour appointment is in an effort to get patients back to functioning according to his podcast. Unfortunately, there is no mention of them assessing patients' temporomandibular joint. Doctors leave that up to dentists There is no dentist as part of their pain management team. Dr Felix Liao D.D.S. would be a major asset to this assessment team.

Medical Treatment of Fibromyalgia

Medications - antidepressants, muscle relaxants, pain pills, anti-inflammatory pills, sleeping pills etc.

Medical modalities - include tai chi, massage, transcutaneous electrical nerve stimulation T.E.N. (ie Dr Ho's machine on TV) , acupuncture, ultrasound, trigger point injections, physical therapy, myofascial release, spray and stretch technique, laser, moist heat, cold treatment ,occupational therapy, psychiatric assessment, biofeedback training, relaxation, meditation and nutrition.

The doctors make it clear that there is no known medical cure for fibromyalgia.

While this seems to be the prevailing opinion of the medical community, I refer you to Mary Catherine Aarssen, from chapter 1. At the time of the initial interview, she had her fibromyalgia symptoms for 36 years and she saw medical doctors without any significant improvement. Following her treatment with Dr Brock Rondeau, a TMJ dentist , she experienced significant relief. Her letter to the press regarding her fibromyalgia and dental treatment can be found in chapter 1.

The treatment of fibromyalgia is a challenge in the field of medicine, however Dr Gole, who is a Head Neck and Facial Pain Dentist in Hasting Michigan and Dr Brock Rondeau , a dentist in London, Ontario are having success in treating fibromyalgia symptoms. Dentists cannot advertise that they can help fibromyalgia symptoms as it is a medical diagnosis. When the dentist treats the TMJ dysfunction and teeth alignment the fibromyalgia symptoms often improve.

I have interviewed many people with fibromyalgia using the TMJ questionnaire that I got from my TMJ manual when I took the certified TMJ Course by the Academy of Head Neck and Facial Pain in Houston Texas. They all have TMJ dysfunction.

Several of the women that I interviewed have already gone to Dr Brock Rondeau, a TMJ dentist and have a dental splint to reposition their jaw, not just a night guard. Many of their fibromyalgia symptoms have improved dramatically and they are now sleeping through the night. The splint is only Phase I of their treatment.

In Phase II the dentist must stabilize the bite in the correct position by orthodontics (braces, crown and bridges, or an overlay denture, partial or complete dentures).

When both of these treatment steps are followed, most patients are relieved of many if not most of their fibromyalgia symptoms.

Chapter 3

The Link Between Fibromyalgia and TMJ Temporomandibular Joint

He who has health, has hope;
and he who has hope has everything.
~ Thomas Carlyle

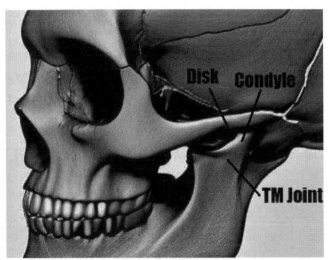

Illustration by Diana Wisemen

The temporomandibular joint is formed by the connection of the lower jaw with the upper jaw. **Note the placement of the disc, TMJ, and condyle.** You may need to refer to the diagram on the previous page as you read this chapter. Everybody has two TMJ (temporomandibular joints). In this chapter TMJ and TMJ dysfunction may be interchanged as people are not familiar with the term TMJD.

In order for this chapter to have a greater impact, I invite everyone with fibromyalgia and/or TMJ to do the self-examination, and TMJ questionnaire that follows. We will be exploring exactly what TMJ is, and how TMJ and fibromyalgia may be interrelated.

Self-examination for TMJ:

A TMJ self-exam is very easy to perform and can be conducted in just a few moments.

Dr Wesley E. Shankland, a TMJ dentist gives the following instruction for TMJ self-exam:

Jaw movements: Looking directly into a wall mirror, slowly open and close your mouth. Watch to see if your jaw moves in a straight line or if it seems to move to one side or the other. Watch this movement both as you open and close your jaw.

With a normal, uninjured temporomandibular joint, the lower jaw should move in a straight line both when opening and when closing. With your mouth open, you should be able to get three fingers between your upper and lower jaw.

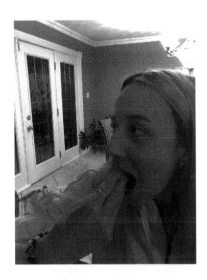

With your mouth open just a little, move your jaw to the left and right. The sideways movements should be about the same in each direction. Lastly, move your lower jaw forward. You should be able to bring the lower jaw forward in a straight line. If any of these movements do not appear to be normal then you might have a problem with your temporomandibular joint.

Listen for TMJ noises: In a quiet room, open and close your mouth several times. Do you hear any type of noise? You should be listening for a popping or clicking sound. You might even hear a crunching or crepitation sound. If you hear a noise, once again look in the mirror and notice if the lower jaw moves or deviates to one side when opening as the noise is heard. If you can hear any of these noises, you might have a TMJ problem.

Pain: Do you experience pain when opening your mouth very wide, side to side or during the forward movement of your jaw? Place your fingers over your TMJ, located just in front of your ears, and apply gentle pressure. Do you notice any tenderness in either or both of your joints? If you place your fingers in your ear canal and gently push forward does your TMJ's hurt?

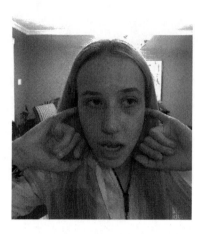

Do your temporomandibular joints hurt when you close hard on your back teeth and squeeze? If so, does placing a tissue between your back teeth and repeating the movement stop the pain? Any of these activities that produce pain should alert you to the possibility of a TMJ problem. Remember: Normal joints do not hurt.

Push on your face: Look in the mirror and push firmly on all the muscles in your face and along your lower jaw. Healthy muscles do not hurt. If you notice a tender area, this may indicate soreness caused by TMJ.

Feel your neck and upper back muscles: Firmly push against the muscles of your neck and upper back. Are there tender spots? If you sit at a computer, or a typewriter or work as a painter or hairstylist, you may experience some discomfort in these areas, as an occupational hazard and this may not be a TMJ problem. Feel your neck where your neck meets your shoulders, and feel the muscles along your shoulders. Are there tender areas? Again, normally healthy muscles are not generally tender. Tender areas in these muscles may indicate a TMJ issue.

A few positive findings may be normal, especially if you're a middle-age to older, or if you work in careers that require overhead arm work, or computer/desk work An inability to open wide enough for at least 2 1/2 fingers to be placed between your front teeth, a significant deviation to one side while opening your mouth, pain, joint noise and numerous tender areas in the facial and neck muscles are all specific symptoms of TMJ. A couple of these symptoms plus suffering from undiagnosed head, neck or facial pain, are possible signs of a developing profile for future TMJ complications.

TMJ, It's Many Faces Diagnosis of TMJ and Related Disorders Wesley E. Shankland, II D.D.S, M.S. 1996

Now that you have completed the TMJ self-exam, the next step is to complete the TMJ Questionnaire on the next page, which is courtesy of Dr Brock Rondeau.

Upon completing these two assessments, you will know whether it would be advisable to see a TMJ specialist to be professionally assessed. The information in this chapter will provide you with additional information that allows you to understand TMJD temporomandibular joint dysfunction better.

TMJ HEALTH QUESTIONNAIRE

Name _____   Date _____

CHIEF CONCERN _____

DATE OF ONSET _____

PAIN SYMPTOMS

Do you get headaches?	Y	N	Do you get headaches in the right or left	Y	N
Do you get migraine headaches?	Y	N	temple areas?		
Do you frequently have neck aches or stiff neck muscles?	Y	N	Do you get headaches in the front or back of your head?	Y	N
Have you ever had chronic shoulder or back pain?	Y	N	Do you clench your teeth during the day?	Y	N
Do you have trouble sleeping soundly?	Y	N	Do you clench your teeth at night?	Y	N
Are your jaws tired when you awaken?	Y	N	Do you grind your teeth when asleep?	Y	N
Are your teeth sore when you awaken?	Y	N	When are your pain symptoms the worst?		

Have your wisdom teeth been extracted?   Y   N

Does anything make you feel better? _____

What medications, if any, are you taking? _____

How often do you take medication for relief of pain?

TRAUMA OR ACCIDENTS

Have you ever had a severe blow to the head or jaw?	Y	N	Have you ever been involved in any serious accidents, such as a car accident?	Y	N
Any whiplash neck injuries?	Y	N	Details _____		

JAW JOINT SYMPTOMS

Does your jaw feel tired after a big meal?	Y	N	Do you feel or hear a 'clicking', 'popping' or 'cracking' noise from either jaw joint?	Y	N
Are there any foods you avoid eating?	Y	N			
Do you ever get dizzy?	Y	N	Has your jaw ever locked when you were unable to open or close?	Y	N
Do you ever feel faint?	Y	N			
Do you ever feel nauseated?	Y	N	Do you have difficulty opening wide or yawning?	Y	N
Is there a family history of jaw joint (TMJ) problems or headaches?	Y	N	Have you ever had pain in either jaw joint?	Y	N
			Does your jaw ache when you open wide?	Y	N

EAR AND EYE SYMPTOMS

Do you have pain in either ear?	Y	N	Do you wear glasses or contacts?	Y	N
Do you suffer from any loss of hearing?	Y	N	Are there times when your eyesight blurs?	Y	N
Do you have itchiness or stuffiness in either ear?	Y	N	Do you get pain in, around or behind either eye?	Y	N
Do you hear ringing, buzzing, or hissing sounds in either ear?	Y	N			

BREATHING

Do you have allergies?	Y	N	Is your nose stuffed when you don't have a cold?	Y	N
Do you have sinus problems?	Y	N	Have you been diagnosed with Sleep Apnea?	Y	N
Do you snore at night?	Y	N	Have you had a sleep study done at a Sleep Clinic (hospital)?	Y	N

Rev.03/20/09

Courtesy of Dr. Brock Rondeau

What Are Temporomandibular Joints?

According to dental books, the temporomandibular joint (TMJ) is the most complex joint in the human body. The jaw joints are complex hinges that connect the lower jaw, or mandible, to the skull. They are made up of bones, ligaments, muscles, cartilage, and fascia. You have one on each side of your jaw.

The TMJ and Airway Connection:

According to the American TMJ Association booklet of Washington U.S.A. 1998, eating, speaking and breathing all depend upon the jaw and TMJ. The TMJ is the temporomandibular joint, more commonly referred to as the jaw joint. It is located in front of the ear and is used in jaw movement.

Millions of people suffer from head, neck, and facial pain without knowing the cause. Millions more experience problems with snoring and sleep apnea, causing sleepiness during the day. Panic attacks, dizziness, memory loss and weight problems often affect these same people. The search for help is difficult, many are told that they are simply not dealing well with stress, or that it is "all in your head." As they go from doctor to doctor, some will endure surgery in an attempt to reduce pain and find relief.

TMJ problems have been treated by dentists for many years. Breathing problems such as Obstructive Sleep Apnea (OSA) have also been treated by dentists working together with physicians for many years. The connection between these conditions have previously been overlooked. This created a gap in treatment for those who suffered these conditions, until recently.

TMJ and the Muscular-Skeletal Link:

The most frequent problem experienced in TMJ is displacement of the disc from between the lower jaw and the socket of the skull (as seen in diagram on page 33), which may worsen over time. If the disc locks out of place and limits mouth opening, one can eventually develop arthritis of the jaw joint. Head, neck and facial pain is a frequent result of TMJ problems. Pain and dysfunction of the jaw often causes headaches. This is one of the most common TMJ symptoms. The TMJ headache usually causes pain in the temples, as well as frequently behind the eye and at the base of the skull. This headache pain may be so severe that it is often mistaken for and initially diagnosed as either a migraine headache or a headache caused by the neck and postural problems. Further exploration is often warranted, as they often occur with TMJ dysfunction.

Other Symptoms of TMJ Problems:

In his book <u>TMJ The Self Help Program,</u> -John Toddley (Constant Schrader and James Dillon 1990), as well as the TMJ associate book, he outlines following additional symptoms:

- Pain in the ear or in the TMJ
- Tenderness of the jaw muscle
- Clicking or popping of the jaw
- Difficulty mouth opening or chewing
- Headaches, sometimes severe
- Ringing in the ear
- Hearing loss
- Sinus pain and dizziness
- Noise in the jaw

If you have fibromyalgia or TMJ how many of these symptoms pertain to you?

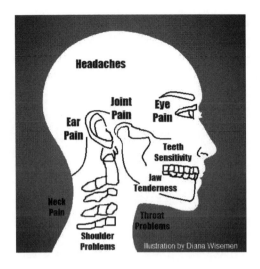

As you can see in the diagram above, if your jaw is back or misaligned, it will affect your neck and jaw joint, as well as create other problems identified as in the diagram above. This is the position that your bite should be in. If you have TMJD, the condyle may be pushed back, causing pressure on the nerves and blood vessels in your jaw. This displacement can cause your muscles to be in spasm which causes ear, eye, throat, headaches symptoms etc.

The Upper Airway - The Primary Use for the Jaw:

The most common problem seen in the upper airway is the narrowing of the airway by the tongue. As the tongue relaxes, it will fall back, reducing or totally blocking the breathing tube, particularly at night. This is why I, and many others, wear a splint at night to keep the lower jaw pulled forward. Large tonsils, enlarged soft palate or uvula and excess fatty tissue can also cause reductions to the upper airway. The tongue forms the front of the upper airway and attaches to the lower jaw. Moving the lower jaw forward or backwards will increase or decrease the airway. The muscles of the lower jaw automatically position the jaw and allow breathing. When the demand on the jaw muscles exceeds their capacity, muscular pain and dysfunction occurs.

These excessive demands of the jaw muscles can be responsible for TMJ problems.

The upper airway is a muscular structure. Conditions that lead to muscular problems of the jaw or neck may lead to problems in the upper airway. Forward posturing of the jaw or neck, as well as a forward head posture may also lead to problems in the upper airway and are similarly linked with TMJ complications.

Upper Airway Symptoms The Source of TMJ Symptoms:

According to the TMJ Association booklet, the most severe upper airway problem is Obstructive Sleep Apnea (OSA). This is a serious condition that occurs with posture breakdown and requires medical diagnosis and management. Accurate diagnosis of this condition must be made in a sleep clinic and will be discussed in the next chapter on sleep.

Less severe upper airway problems may be associated with a variety of symptoms including the following:

- Frequent night-time awakening
- Startled and disorientation upon awakening
- Stomach acid reflux and heartburn
- Snoring and loud night-time breathing
- Disturbing dreams
- Chest wall soreness
- Morning headaches
- Frequent nausea
- Gagging easily on food or pills
- Unexplained weight gain or loss
- Falling asleep easily
- Grogginess and dizziness
- Short term memory loss

If you have been diagnosed with fibromyalgia or TMJ, how many of these symptoms pertain to you?

TMJ Airway Treatment:

Specific dental appliances are required to treat TMJ airway challenges. The devices are designed to move the lower jaw forward and elevate the tongue. This allows freer breathing and relaxes the jaw muscles. If the upper palate is narrow, the palate may need expanding. This will be discussed in further detail later in this chapter as well as the chapter on sleep. The TMJ related pain problems can then begin to resolve. Postural changes automatically begin, as the forward head posture is no longer needed to maintain the airway. Most people find that they stand taller, experience a reduction in pain, sleepiness and find significant resolution with any other problems they may be experiencing.

There are significant differences in treatment style between the dental and medical communities: TMJ dentists generally use splints to reposition the jaw or expand the palate allowing for the alleviation of many jaw, head and neck problems. Medical doctors typically treat TMJ with medication such as pain pills, muscle relaxants, antidepressants, and a variety of other pharmaceuticals. Medical modalities such as ultrasound, T.E.N.S. (transcutaneous electrical nerve stimulation), physical therapy, moist hot or cold treatment, massage, acupuncture, biofeedback, meditation, tai chi, exercise, infrared, laser, stretching and analgesic sprays are also used. These treatments help the pain but do not alleviate the underlying problem, and are not effective over the long term.

Other Ways that the TMJ Joints Get Damaged:

When I took my TMJ Assistant Course in Texas I was taught that there are two ways that the temporomandibular joint can be damaged:

- Accidental trauma
- Micro-trauma

Accidental trauma can occur in many different ways: A blow to the jaw in a fall or other accidents can stretch and tear the ligaments surrounding the joint. When this occurs, the disc begins to slip, and causes clicking or popping. An extremely common accidental injury which can trigger a TMJ injury is whiplash, often associated with car accidents. Many of the people I interviewed with fibromyalgia had whiplash or a head injury of some kind. A displaced disc in the jaw can occur if someone has an incident of respiratory distress. The jaw gets over extended when the patient is unconscious and intubated in order to assist their breathing. When I interviewed patients with fibromyalgia, I only interviewed two men: both men had been intubated during a respiratory emergency. One of my interviewees, a woman, remembered that her jaw started clicking after she had her wisdom teeth removed. Had her mouth been opened too wide displacing the disc? Many of the people that were interviewed with fibromyalgia had whiplash or had some other kind of accident. I personally went head first off my bike as a young girl. A mother I met at the fibromyalgia conference, said her daughter's fibromyalgia symptoms started when she flew off her bike and knocked out her two front teeth.

According to Dr Moles, a dentist, **micro-trauma** can occur because of the structure of the face. Very simply, when the teeth and/or the jaws do not properly align, undesirable twisting, torquing and pulling forces will be applied to the joints every time the teeth come into contact. Treatment of micro trauma is eliminating or reducing any improper alignment by correcting crooked teeth or improperly aligned jaw structure. A tooth which is significantly out of position will not be there to support the bite. When a tooth is too high it will cause the jaw to tip, placing undesirable torque and load on the joint. Any time the temporomandibular joint (TMJ) is not in the proper position one will have muscle spasm and pain not only in the face and the neck muscles but can continue downward affecting the rest of the body.

The Role of Teeth in TMJ:

Between the two temporomandibular joints is a double arch of your upper and lower teeth. The teeth have a profound influence on the position of the ball (condyle) in the jaw socket as well as the amount of stress placed on the joint. According to Dr. Taddey, when the bite between the teeth is not stable, the resulting slight movements or displacement within the joint, repeated each day, may wear down the disc, eventually producing bone-on-bone contact and TMJ damage. Jaw pain can come from stretched ligaments, and inflammation in the nerve-rich tissue in the jaw or muscles. Normal muscles do not have trigger points. Healthy muscles have no taunt bands or muscle fibers and are not tender when palpated. Even when resolved, Dr Taddey, in his book TMJ The Self Help Program, suggests that trigger points may remain in the muscles for as long as ten or twenty years. To illustrate, if we recall Mary Catherine Aarsen in Chapter 1. She had been diagnosed with fibromyalgia, and had been experiencing symptoms for 36 years before she had treatment for her TMJ. Once her TMJ was treated, many of her fibromyalgia symptoms began to resolve.

Effect of Missing Teeth on TMJ

Missing back teeth:

Again, according to Dr. Taddy, in his book, back teeth support the temporomandibular joint and are important to its movement. Jaws stay correctly positioned when teeth and jaw muscles work together. The muscles pull up on the jaw, and the back teeth and wisdom teeth keep the jaw placed correctly. When those teeth are missing, the unopposed upward pull of the muscles drives the ball (condyle) deeply in the socket, which can cause TMJ problems. Wear on the back teeth can also create uneven pull and pressure, is another cause of TMJ problems.

Missing Teeth Causing Abnormal Load on the Jaw:

A more serious problem occurs when tooth material is lost on one side of the jaw. In such cases, the lack of symmetry increases the potential for torquing, twisting or other damaging forces to be generated in the joint on the opposite side, thereby injuring cartilage and ligaments.

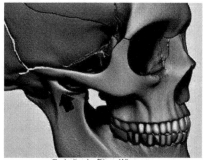
Illustration by Diana Wisemen

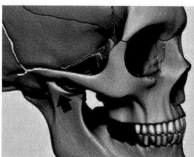
Illustration by Diana Wisemen

Effect of Malocclusion (A Bad Bite) on TMJ:

Malocclusion may be produced by poor development of the jaw, or the removal of teeth. When removed teeth are not replaced, the pull of muscles on the jaw can cause TMJ. Malocclusion may also be caused by a high dental restoration, a poorly fitting denture or partial denture or disc displacement.

In addition to TMJ, this misalignment can cause bruxism: When a bite is misaligned, the brain tends to make a person grind his or her teeth to even the bite, thus reducing the malocclusion. This becomes a vicious cycle: Malocclusion produces bruxism: Bruxism produces sore muscles and sensitive teeth; and sore muscles and sensitive teeth can produce malocclusion.

Effect of Bruxism on TMJ:

Bruxism is an abnormal grinding of the teeth. If grinding continues or develops later in life, TMJ may develop. Bruxism usually occurs during sleep. Dr Felix Liao indicates this is due to one trying to open their airway causing grinding of their teeth. **(Six Foot Tiger, Three Foot Cage)**. One indication that a person is a bruxer is sore jaw muscles when waking in the morning. Bruxing produces muscle pain, sensitivity, and worn teeth.

Effect of Clenching on TMJ:

Clenching is a form of bruxism that can also cause TMJ. Clenching may occur at any time. However, it is most noticeable during times of frustration, concentration or stress.

Effect of Being Double-Jointed on TMJ:

People who are double-jointed suffer from a problem termed ligament laxity. Women are more commonly diagnosed with ligament laxity, because women have a hormone that is released from their pituitary gland : relaxin, which helps in the birth of children. Is this why many women begin to experience TMJ symptoms after they give birth? Ligament laxity is a fairly common problem in active young women who suffer with TMJ.

TMJ Its Many Faces Wesley E Shankland D.D.S M.S 1996 (dentist)

Other causes of TMJ dysfunction:

According to Dr Brock Rondeau DDS, in his <u>Diagnosis and Treatment of TMJ Manual</u> (2020), there are other things that can cause TMJ problems:

1. When the lower jaw is too far back in relation to the upper jaw, the distal tip of the lower jaw (condyle) becomes posteriorly displaced. This causes the disc to be displaced anteriorly, when the patient is in a proper bite. The clicking is caused by a displaced disc.

2. Constricted maxillary arch - high palate on the roof of the mouth- which causes the distal tip of the lower jaw to become posteriorly displaced.

3. Forward head posture.

4. Intubation procedures in hospitals can cause dislocation of the jaw. It is recommended by many TMJ sources, that people who suffer with TMJ should request nasal intubation, so the jaw is not affected.

Musical Instruments and TMJ:

Certain musical instruments can contribute to, and aggravate TMJ dysfunction. The clarinet has a mouthpiece that goes between the lingual of the upper incisors and the labial of the lower incisors causing the mandible and the distal tip of the lower jaw (condyle) to go posteriorly. This can cause a compression of the nerves and blood vessels distal to the tip of the lower jaw (condyle).

Crossbite and TMJ:

When the middle of the top teeth and the middle of the bottom teeth do not line up, this is a condition referred to as crossbite. The next photo is Danielle. She has been diagnosed with both fibromyalgia and TMJ dysfunction. I met her when I was doing interviews with individuals with cross diagnoses. She is in a crossbite and her bottom teeth deviated to the right, as displayed in this photo. She also hears a clicking in her jaw on her right side. For Danielle, this crossbite is her present bite. This type of problem can also occur as a result of incorrect or inappropriate treatment. I was in a crossbite when my bridge was on incorrectly.

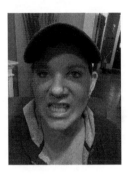

Treatment of TMJ by TMJ Dentists

According Dr Brock Rondeau, in his *Diagnosis and Treatment of TMJ Manual* (2020):

Phase 1: Diagnostic phase; 4-6 months:

The objective of phase 1 is to **reduce the signs and symptoms** of TMJ dysfunction, improve the range of motion of the lower jaw, reduce the muscle spasms, recapture anteriorly displaced discs in the jaw, and establish a normal disc-condyle relationship, finding the correct position of the jaw.

The most common treatment for temporomandibular disorders is the use of repositioning orthotics, commonly called splints. These devices are made from a number of different materials and are fabricated in a number of different shapes, forms and sizes: Splints may fit on the upper teeth, the lower teeth or both upper and lower depending on what is required to address the concerns identified. There are many types of splints but all share the following goals: **realigning the joint, muscle relaxation and postural change.**

Realigning the Joint: This is often accomplished by creating and fitting a plastic, molded splint which is designed to fit over either the upper or lower teeth. Then interdental space has indentations into which the opposing set of teeth can fit. The dentist creates these in order to guide the patient's lower jaw gently into a new position every time it closes. Note: This is not a flat plane splint that most regular dentists order, which do not reposition the jaw.

Muscle Relaxation: By placing a plastic plate over one's set of teeth, the protective signals traveling from the roots of the teeth to the brain and then to the facial muscles are interrupted. Shaping the plastic plate adjusts positioning of the jaw, prevents the muscles from putting excessive stress on the jaw joints, reducing muscle strain.

Postural Change: The lower jaw is attached to the base of the skull by ligaments and muscles. Guiding the jaw into a new position will create contraction or stretch in these muscles. When the length of a muscle changes, it affects all of the surrounding muscles. To see the effects of changing the position of the lower jaw and therefore, the surrounding muscles, try a simple experiment: Jut your lower jaw forward as far as possible and then move your head back over your spine. Notice how the tension in the muscles under your chin relaxes. By moving the lower jaw, the dentist can affect the posture of the head upon the spinal column, thereby affecting the tension and dynamics of the neck muscles. Placing an orthotic device between the teeth will change the centre of gravity of the head, affecting the tension on the face and neck muscles. My dental splint brought my jaw forward, relieved the spasm in my jaw, and my neck, which improved my posture, leading to relief from my headaches.

Some important thoughts for splint wearers: An important consideration when approaching splint therapy, is that the success or failure of the therapy, depends on the commitment of the patient. It is **absolutely** imperative for you to follow the dentist's instructions to the letter. It may not be comfortable, or convenient, but if those instructions are not followed, the chance of complete resolution is greatly diminished. For example, I had to wear my double dental splint 24 hours a day, except to brush my teeth. I did this for six months and could only eat soft food, and could not take it out even for a few bites of food. The splint also affected my speech, but I knew if I wanted to get better I was going to follow the dentist's instructions and leave my splint in place.

Phase II Treatment Phase:

The objective of Phase II is to **alter the bite** (occlusion) so when the teeth contact in the centric occlusion (a good bite), the tip of the jaw bone (condyle) is the correct position in the jaw joint. This can be accomplished with orthodontic and restorative treatment.

Orthodontics: A combination of jaw stabilization appliances and straight wire orthodontics are used to approximate the upper and lower teeth in a position where the TM joints are stable. In my case, I had braces for 1 1/2 years to stabilize my jaw in the proper position, and had a partial denture where my teeth were missing from where my bridge was removed.

Crown and Bridge: In cases where the spaces between the posterior teeth are minimal and the posterior teeth are heavily restored, badly broken down or when placed in order to approximate the upper and lower teeth to hold the position where the TM joints are stable.

Overlay Partial: In cases where there are a large number of posterior teeth missing, overlay partials may be the treatment of choice. Overlay partials are also a viable option when the patient needs something more permanent to stabilize the jaw and cannot afford either orthodontics or crowns or bridges.

A non-appliance treatment that some dentists use is to inject botox. This is a drug which is used to treat TMJD. Botox works by paralysing the over used masseter muscle in the jaw. When these muscles are unable to move, they can no longer fire extreme force. This prohibits the muscles from getting their regular workout, allowing them to rest, and giving them time to heal and to repair themselves. During the resting phase, symptoms of TMJ are relieved. The benefits of Botox therapy typically last up to 5 months depending on severity of condition. It can be expensive, however. At one dental office the cost was $1100 per treatment. It is important, when considering treatment options, that although Botox treatments relieve muscle spasm temporarily, it is not a long term solution to TMJD. This treatment does not solve the structural problem of a narrow upper palate that some TMJD patients present with.

If you have fibromyalgia or have been diagnosed with TMJ, the information so far may have you considering that there may be other avenues of treatment that you may want to explore to give you some relief of your pain. The input of a specialised TMJ dentist cannot be underestimated. After reading many TMJ books written by dentists, I discovered that there is a chapter on fibromyalgia in a good majority of them. How come more people do not know this fact? I am a nurse and had no idea that there might even be a connection. That is one of the reasons I started my quest for more knowledge. I read many TMJ books, took the American Academy of Head, Neck and Facial Pain Certified TMJ Assistant Course, even though I did not want to work in a dentist's office, I want to learn more about the structural and mechanical aspects of the jaw. I have interviewed a great many people with TMJ dysfunction. This information was invaluable in my crusade to understand how fibromyalgia and TMJ are connected.

Chapter 4

Airway and Sleep

Sleep is that golden chain that ties health and our bodies together.
~ Thomas Dekker

How Does Lack of Sleep Affect Fibromyalgia?

According to the Mayo Clinic's website, signs and symptoms of myofascial pain syndrome may make it difficult to sleep at night. Individuals who have this disorder, may have trouble finding a comfortable sleep position, and often any change in position may stimulate a trigger point causing the person to awaken.

One study found that 99 percent of fibromyalgia patients suffered from poor sleep quality. This in turn influenced the severity of physical pain, fatigue and difficulty with social functioning. In addition to restless, unrefreshing sleep, and insomnia, people with fibromyalgia are more likely to suffer from other sleep disorders. Recent research found obstructive sleep apnea present in 1/2 of the group of fibromyalgia patients.

Although airway was discussed in the TMJ chapter, I felt it was important to reiterate that the airway and sleep are related. Several of these issues will therefore be repeated.

Obstructive sleep apnea can be addressed by TMJ Dentists or Airway Mouth Dentists They can also assess for narrow palate, overbite, and a bottom jaw that is posteriorly displaced, causing the tongue to be too far back, creating a compromised airway.

Relationship between sleep disorders and temporomandibular joint (TMJ) dysfunction:

Dr. Brock Rondeau believes that anyone who enters dentistry, does so with a strong desire to help people achieve a higher level of health. Dental school curricula emphasise treating teeth and gums. They are not, however, taught how to diagnose temporomandibular joint dysfunction, snoring, or obstructive sleep apnea.

In his experience, rather than using a traditional tooth and gum dentistry, of making room for all the permanent teeth: to extract bicuspid teeth and retract the six front teeth. removing these crowded teeth, and significantly reduces the width of the smile, and closes the airway, moves the tongue back, and increases the future risk of snoring and obstructive sleep apnea.

Mouth breathing causes constriction of the upper arch, as the tongue does not expand the upper arch when the patient swallows incorrectly, up to 2000 times a day. This constriction of the upper arch causes the lower jaw to fall back, causing two major health problems:

1. When the lower jaw goes back, the tongue also goes back and can obstruct the airway particularly when the patient sleeps on their back, and can increase the severity of life-threatening obstructive sleep apnea.
2. When the lower jaw goes back due to mouth breathing, it increases the incidence of jaw joint problems: When the lower jaw goes back, the top of the lower jaw goes back too far and impinges on the nerves and blood/vessels in front of the ear, causing tinnitus, fainting, dizziness, and back problems.

Lower Positioning Splint

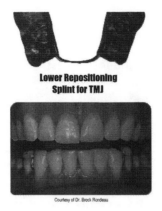

**Lower Repositioning
Splint for TMJ**

Courtesy of Dr. Brock Rondeau

Treatment (by Dr Brock Rondeau):

The treatment would be to fabricate a lower splint that moves the lower jaw forward away from the nerves and blood vessels. This lower splint is worn on the lower teeth all day long, even when eating. This treatment significantly reduces the pain symptoms of TMD temporomandibular dysfunction.

It is important to remember whatever technique is being used to treat orthodontic problems, TMD or snoring, and sleep apnea you must be aware of the importance of increasing the size of the nasal and pharyngeal airway

His observation is that patients with deep overbites (upper teeth overlapping the lower teeth) frequently have TMD (temporal mandibular dysfunction) symptoms, particularly in females over the age of 20. Also patients with underdeveloped lower jaw seem to have the majority of jaw joint TMD problems. I would urge readers to be aware of this and if the TMD symptoms persist to get treated as soon as possible because TMD is a progressive condition that frequently gets worse over time.

He strongly believe that all patients should be screened for obstructive sleep apnea and TMD and if the dentist is not qualified to treat, should refer these patients to a dentist that is, because as I stated at the onset, we all went into practice with the strong desire to help improve the quality of the life of our patients.

(End of article) by Dr Brock Rondeau dentist.

Although sleep problems have not always been considered a key component of fibromyalgia, today, sleep problems are recognized as a central characteristic of fibromyalgia. It is estimated that 50 % of people with fibromyalgia have sleep apnea. The presence of disrupted sleep, as well as the lack of restorative sleep and daytime fatigue are now commonly used as markers to diagnose the disorder. These are frequently present, along with physical pain issues, and mood and cognitive symptoms.

Nearly all people with fibromyalgia experience some form of sleep problems. Poor sleep contributes to a wide range of challenges mentally, and physically. Daily functioning is also often impacted. Sleep deficits also often exacerbate other fibromyalgia symptoms. One study found that 99% of fibromyalgia patients suffered poor sleep quality. This was found to influence how severely they experience physical pain, fatigue, and difficulty with social functioning. It is also reported that poor sleep lowers pain thresholds, making people more sensitive to pain.

Do you have an impaired mouth and airway? Discover your holistic mouth score by Dr Felix Liao, an Airway Mouth Dentist. This self-survey begins to illuminate how the mouth's structure and architecture contributes to medical, dental, and mental-emotional symptoms. This is essentially a checklist of the more common orofacial, dental and body signs and symptoms of an impaired mouth.

The higher the score, the more likely you have been living with an impaired mouth for a long time. You can access and download the digital versions of the following templates and materials at http://holisticmouthsolutions.com

Impaired Mouth Syndrome Score

Courtesy of Dr. Felix Liao, DDS, Author of Six-foot Tiger, Three-foot Cage

Mouth	Score	Body	Score
Snoring, morning dry mouth	0 1	Gasping or choking in sleep	0 1
Teeth grinding, jaw clenching	0 1	Neck, shoulder, or back pain; headaches	0 1
Mouth breathing, chapped lips	0 1	Erectile dysfunction or PMS	0 1
Persistent/wandering dental sensitivity	0 1	High blood pressure, heart disease	0 1
Gum recession and/or redness	0 1	Diabetes type 2, bloating after meals	0 1
Clicking/locking jaw joints, zigzag jaw opening	0 1	Weight gain, pot belly; acid reflux	0 1
Morning headache and/or sore jaws	0 1	Daytime sleepiness, fatigue	0 1
Deep overbite or underbite (weak chin)	0 1	Senile memory, ADD/ADHD	0 1
Frequent cavities or broken/chipped teeth	0 1	Frequent colds, flu, and skin disorders	0 1
Teeth prints on the sides of the tongue	0 1	Obstructive sleep apnea from a sleep test	0 1
Bony outgrowth on palate or inside lower jaw	0 1	Stuffy/runny nose, scratchy/itchy throat	0 1
Sunken lips and reverse smile curve (sad)	0 1	Forward head: ears ahead of shoulders	0 1
History of teeth extractions for braces	0 1	Waking up to urinate more than once	0 1
Bulge under lower jaw, double chin	0 1	Large neck size (M>17, W>15)	0 1
History of lots of dental work + medical symptoms	0 1	Poor digestion and elimination	0 1
Malocclusion (crowded teeth)	0 1	Depression, anxiety, grouchiness	0 1
Total Score		Total Score	

www.HolisticMouthSolutions.com

Individuals who score high on this questionnaire should look for an airway dentist to be assessed.

One thing I have learned after going to Dr Liao's Airway, Mouth Dentist conference, is that these dentists will treat TMJ, recapture the disc in the jaw, expand the upper jaw (maxilla) and also expand the lower jaw (mandible) if measurements indicate it is necessary. A TMJ dentist will treat TMJ by recapturing the disc in the jaw, bringing the lower jaw forward. They may not, however, address the narrow upper jaw (maxilla) or the narrow lower jaw (mandible.) In order to address the entire issue, it is recommended that patients look for an **airway dentist first.** Unfortunately, there are only a limited number in Canada. At the very least, I recommend finding a good TMJ dentist to assess your jaw, so you can be treated.

Dr James Garry (dentist), who researched airway issues and wrote the book Upper Airway Compromise and Musculo-Skeletal Dysfunction of the Head and Neck, identified the following symptoms of upper airway obstruction:

- Chronic open mouth habits
- Lip pursing when swallows
- Facial asymmetry
- Dry lips (usually from chronic mouth breathing)
- Herpetic lesion on lips usually from nocturnal mouth breathing and drooling
- TMJ. noise (popping and crepitus)
- Bruxism
- Cervical Erosion
- Headaches in the frontal, temporal, and occipital region
- Dysphagia (difficulty swallowing) due to a lack of volume for the tongue within the dental arches as a result of early airway obstruction from enlarged tonsils, adenoids, and or nasal blockage
- Open bite
- High or narrow upper palate (roof of the mouth)
- Scalloped tongue (tooth prints on border of the tongue due to lack of intra-oral volume for the tongue)
- Chewing cheek

- Dry mouth in the morning (due to mouth breathing during the night)
- Drooling during sleep (open mouth)
- Enlarged tonsils or adenoids
- Constantly tired (anemia and low oxygen)
- Bloodshot eyes
- Chronic earaches
- Chronic recurrent throat infections
- Obstructive sleep apnea
- Hyperactivity
- Severe fatigue after exercise
- Constantly tired
- Tinnitus (ringing in the ear)
- Fullness in the ears
- Difficulty in nasal breathing
- Lisping
- Postural problems (forward head posture, side bending of head)
- Edema below the eyes
- Marginal upper lid eczema
- Enuresis (bed wetting) due to nocturnal arousals as a result of a drop in blood oxygen saturation)

If you have fibromyalgia, it may serve you well to record which of these symptoms that you are experiencing:

In my experience, I had lips pursing with swallowing, dry lips, bruxism, difficulty swallowing, scalloped tongue, drooling at night, chronic throat infections, constantly tired , snoring, and forward head posture which caused my shoulder to roll forward. These symptoms went away when Dr Gole took my dental bridge off. It had been sitting too close to the side of my cheek. He said I was in a crossbite. My tongue was blocking my airway, as it was a muscle trying to pull my jaw back into the right position. Once my tongue went back to the normal position I started to sleep better and no longer fell asleep during the day, as I had when I took my CPR instructors course, falling asleep for 10 minutes, twice during the morning, without knowing it.

The Epworth Sleepiness Scale (ESS) is another self-test that can be used to assess sleep quality. It was developed and validated by Dr. Murray Johns of Melbourne, Australia. This is a simple, self-administered questionnaire— widely used by sleep professionals in quantifying the level of daytime sleepiness.

How likely are you to doze off or fall asleep in the following situations, in contrast to feeling 'just tired'? This refers to your usual way of life at present and in the recent past. Use the following scale below, choose the most appropriate number for each situation:

SITUATION CHANCE OF DOZING
0 = would **never** doze
1 = **slight** chance of dozing
2 = **moderate** chance of dozing
3 = **high** chance of dozing

- *Sitting and reading*
- *Watching television*
- *Sitting, inactive in a public place (e.g. theatre, meeting)*
- *As a passenger in a car for an hour without a break*
- *Lying down to rest in the afternoon when circumstances permit Sitting and talking to someone*
- *Sitting quietly after lunch without alcohol*
- *In a car, while stopped for a few minutes in traffic*

TOTAL SCORE:
- the average score is 4 to 8
- my score was 15
- **What is your score?**

The Epworth Sleepiness Scale. http://epworthsleepinessscale.com/about-the-ess/ as seen on page 60.

If I had taken the *Epworth Sleepiness* scale I would have scored a 15: this is very high. My tongue was blocking my airway because I was in a crossbite due to my dental bridge being on incorrectly. I also had an overbite.

Note: If you have an overbite and your mandible (lower jaw) is back, so is your tongue. If you have a narrow or high upper palate your tongue does not fit in your mouth properly. Both can cause airway problems and affect your ability to have a good night's sleep.

Three of the ladies with fibromyalgia that I interviewed in Lakeland, Florida had a CAT scan at the **Breathe Well Sleep Well Clinic** at Clearwater Florida. Two of the ladies had a narrow upper palate, and both experienced sleep apnea. They were fitted with a Vivos splint to expand their upper palate so they could breathe easier. (vivos.com) The other lady was told that she had severe TMJ with bone degeneration and she was referred to Dr Ralph Garcia a TMJ dentist in Tampa. (www.tmjtampabay.com) He made her a splint that brought her bottom jaw forward which increased her airway. Her comment after getting the splint was "Oh my God, I can breathe easier now."

These are only two of the types of splint that can be used to expand the upper or lower palate: the Vivos splint at vivos.com and the DNA (day night time appliance) at www.HolisticMouthSolutions.com.

I interviewed a lady with fibromyalgia and TMJD (temporomandibular joint dysfunction) who has an extremely narrow upper palate (roof of her mouth.) When I measured her upper palate I could only get ½ a cotton roll in her high upper palate. A normal palate accommodates a whole cotton roll. Her tongue did not fit in her mouth properly, causing sleep apnea. She did not sleep well and also had a diagnosis of bipolar or manic depressive disorder. She has headaches in the frontal lobe every night and tested positive for having a very compromised airway. She was a mouth breather, which was related to her deviated septum. No treatment for her sleep deprivation was wanted at this time.

I have since examined two other women diagnosed with bipolar. They also have very narrow upper palates (roof of their mouth). Are these two diagnoses related? I do not know but I found the correlation interesting. There would have to be an assessment of hundreds of bipolar patients to see if this is consistent. The narrow upper palate can be treated with splint. It is worn on the upper palate to make the palate wider, or longer or increase the vertical space, like the ladies that I interviewed who had gone to The Breath Well Sleep Well Clinic and had a CAT Scan to show their compromised airway.

Why do we need sleep:
www. Sleep foundation.org

Sleep is an essential function that allows the body and mind to recharge, leaving us refreshed and alert when we wake up. Healthy sleep also helps the body remain healthy and prevent diseases. Without enough sleep, the brain can't function properly, impairing the ability to concentrate, think clearly, and process memories.

The Sleep Cycle:

Most adults require between seven to nine hours of nightly sleep. Chronic lack of sleep may indicate a sleep disorder. The internal body clock called a circadian rhythm regulates the sleep cycle, controlling when we feel tired and ready for bed or refreshed and alert. When our eyes are exposed to natural or artificial light, it signals an area in the brain to determine whether it is day or night. This light exposure influences our circadian rhythm. As natural light disappears in the evening, the body releases melatonin, a hormone that induces drowsiness. When the sun rises in the morning, the body will release the hormone known as cortisol from the adrenals, promoting energy and alertness.

STAGES OF SLEEP:

Once we fall asleep, our bodies follow a sleep cycle divided into four stages: The first three stages are non-rapid eye movement (NREM) sleep, and the fourth stage is rapid eye movement (REM) sleep.

Stage 1 NREM (non-rapid eye movement): this first stage marks the transition between wakefulness and sleep. This is considered light sleep. Muscles relax, heart rate, breathing, and eye movement begins to slow down Brain waves also begin to slow. This stage typically lasts several minutes.

Stage 2 NREM (non-rapid eye movement): This sleep stage is characterized by deeper sleep. Heart rate and breathing rates continue slowing down and muscles become even more relaxed. Movements will cease and body temperature will decrease. Apart from some brief moments brain waves will also continue to slow. Stage two is typically the longest of the four sleep stages.

Stage 3 NREM (non-rapid eye movement): This stage plays an important role in making us feel refreshed and alert the next day. Heartbeat, breathing, and brain waves activity will reach their lowest level, and the muscles are extremely relaxed. This stage will be longer in the early part of the sleep cycle, and will decrease throughout the night.

Stage 4 REM (rapid eye movement): The first REM stage will occur about 90 minutes into the sleep cycle. As the name suggests, eyes move back-and-forth rather quickly under the eyelids. Breathing rate, heart rate and blood pressure will begin to increase. Dreaming will typically occur during REM sleep. Arms and legs become paralyzed – it's believed this is intended to prevent us from physically acting out our dreams. The duration of each REM sleep cycle increases as the night progresses. Numerous studies have also linked REM sleep to memory consolidation: the process of converting recently learned experiences into long-term memories. The duration of the capital REM stage decreases as we age, causing us to spend more time in the NREM stages.

These four stages will repeat cyclically throughout the night until we wake up. For most people these cycles last between 90 - 120 minutes.

According to the Cleveland Clinic website: https://my.clevelandclinic.org

People with Fibromyalgia spend less time in deep sleep. Their heightened brain activity appears to keep them in lighter stages of sleep, and they may wake twice as often as people who don't have the condition. Deep, non-REM sleep is essential for the brain and body to repair and refresh at a cellular level. The lack of restorative deep sleep may help to explain the fatigue, physical pain, and "brain fog" that is a characteristic symptom for many people with fibromyalgia.

For some patients with fibromyalgia, sleep apnea can be treated with a CPAP (Continuous Positive Airway Pressure) machine. This machine forces air past the obstructed airway. Many people have been able to discontinue their CPAP treatment when they are fitted with an oral splint to hold their bottom jaw forward, as it also pulls their tongue away from the back of their throat, opening up their airway. Dental splints used to expand one's upper palate (roof of mouth) making more room for one's tongue can also be successful in addressing breathing issues.

Obstructive Sleep Apnea (OSA) Symptoms:

- High blood pressure, stroke
- Heart attack sudden death
- Diabetes, obesity
- GERD: acid reflux
- Lower immunity
- Depression, anxiety
- Brain fog, senile memory
- Accelerated aging
- Chronic pain
- Daytime sleepiness, accidents

- Sleep bruxing (teeth grinding)

JAMA 269, no12 (1993) 1548-1550

According to Dr Felix Liao in his book ***Six Foot Tiger, Three Foot Cage 2017*** (pg 81 to 83) deadly obstructive sleep apnea is undetected 75% of the time. He states that the leading causes of obstructive sleep start in the mouth. When seen during a dental exam by him, he found:

- A lower jaw that is short compared with the upper jaw
- Certain shapes of the palate or airway that causes the airway to be narrower or collapse more easily
- A large neck - seventeen inches or more in men, sixteen inches or more in women
- A large tongue that can fall back and block the airway
- Obesity
- Large tonsils and adenoids in children can block the airway

Daytime sleepiness is a cardinal feature of sleep apnea. Others include waking up tired, jaw clenching, and teeth grinding, which is now called bruxism in sleep medicine. All people with fibromyalgia should be assessed for Obstructive Sleep Apnea. You may be one of the 75% of undetected sleep apnea patients. One of the main symptoms of OSA is snoring.

Snoring is the lay term for obstructive breathing during sleep. The sound of snoring originates from the collapsible part of the airway where there is no rigid support. The musculature may fail to maintain normal tones in the respiratory tract if one consumes alcoholic beverages, sedative-hypnotics tranquillisers, or antihistamines before retiring. Nasal or septal deformity, nasal tumours, and sinusitis with nasal polyps are also causes of snoring.

Dr James Garry (dentist) <u>Upper Airway Compromise and Musculo-Skeletal Dysfunction of the Head and Neck</u> shares that what typically happens during sleep is that all the muscles in the upper body relax. The result is a collapse of the tissues in the upper airway. Most patients have no difficulty breathing while awake but develop prolonged periods of partial airway obstruction with shorter episodes of complete obstruction after they fall asleep.

Common Complaints of the Apneic Patient:

A common complaint of an apneic patient is awakening with a dry mouth and/or a scratchy throat. These patients cannot adequately ventilate themselves during deep stage sleep. They repeatedly rouse themselves to lighter stages of sleep just to breathe. As a result, they do not feel rested upon awakening. Many of these patients may fall asleep while driving an automobile or while working on a job. They fall asleep while watching TV programs, reading or carrying on a conversation. Morning headaches are common as a result of low oxygen saturation, and often have difficulty rousing in the morning. When I had my compromised airway, I would fall asleep watching TV programs, and I could not drive 80 miles to the city without pulling over on the side of the road to have a fifteen minute nap before continuing my journey.

Side Effects of Sleep Apnea:

Behaviour changes have been noted in both children and adults suffering from sleep apnea. The most typical changes are depression and agitation. Intellectual impairment is not uncommon, and one's inability to carry on concentrated study can make it difficult to perform assigned jobs. The dentist that I work with has expanded children's palates only to find that their sleep quality as well as their behaviour improves. On **YouTube,** Dr Ben Miraglia, *Connecting Sleep Disorders, Breathing and ADD/ADHD* highlights the difficulty of identifying differences between sleep deprived children and ADHD children. This **YouTube** video is a must for parents of ADHD children.

Sleep Position and Apnea:

Cartwright et al. found that patients with obstructive sleep apnea associated with supine (lying on back) sleep position had a significant improvement of apneic episodes when they altered their sleep position to sleeping on their side. If a person cannot sleep in any position other than on their back, elevating the head of the bed 30 to 40 degrees, reducing the gravitational pull of the mandible (lower jaw) and tongue, could be an option.

Leg Movement During Sleep:

Dr Ralph A Pascualy, a medical doctor, shared that some 40% of older adults experience involuntary leg movement associated with sleep. Dr Jon Russel, another medical doctor, also states that 16% of people with fibromyalgia also have restless leg syndrome (called nocturnal myoclonus). In restless leg syndrome, the person experiences a tingly feeling and urge to move the legs. This may interfere with falling asleep. They may also experience periodic leg movements, which is expressed as kicking motions that occur repeatedly during sleep. These movements may awaken the sleeper. Even if they do not awaken the sleeper, it can also be more disruptive to the bed partner. If you or your bed partner experience either of these disorders, it would be of great benefit to talk with a sleep specialist about possible treatment options.

Although I do not have sleep apnea, I wear a splint on my upper and lower jaw at night that interlocks and keeps my tongue forward. This has greatly improved my quality of sleep.

It is imperative that the fibromyalgia patients have their airway and their jaw assessed in order to receive treatment that can open their airway and enable them to have quality sleep. Doing this will frequently address many of their symptoms such as brain fog, improve their restless leg syndrome, physical pain, fatigue and irritability.

I would recommend that you read ***Six-foot Tiger, Three-Foot Cage:*** *Take Charge of Your Health by Taking Charge of Your Mouth by Dr Felix Liao which* can be purchased through Amazon.

Here are three reviews of the book **Six-*foot Tiger, Three-Foot Cage*** by medical professionals, found in the front of the book:

"I highly recommend this revolutionary book by Dr Liao because it's time to put an end to the suffering by patients and their families stemming from craniofacial deficiencies. This book connects the dots between underlying etiology and clinical signs and symptoms, and offers both solutions and life stories that illustrate the importance of oral health that support whole body health."
Dr Dave Singh, DDSc,PhD, DMD

"The book is readable for laymen, dentists and other professionals, and makes us all aware of how important oral airways can affect major metabolic and physical abnormalities and finally to disease states. The clarity and simplicity of his arguments are supported by the large body of references for professional corroboration. We should all read this book!"
George Yu Clinical Professor, Medical Research Associates

"As a holistic MD, I often wonder why certain people don't get well despite good diet, supplements, detoxing and attention to their mental/emotional and spiritual health. Dr Felix Liao's book ***Six-Foot Tiger, Three-Foot Cage*** brilliantly explains why. By weaving amazing case studies and compelling research, Dr Liao has written a ground-breaking book that everyone, especially physicians and dentists, should read. I truly believe that this could be the missing piece of the puzzle for sufferers of chronic pain, chronic fatigue, sleep apnea/snoring and much more."
Dr Margaret Gennaro, MD.

PLEASE CONSIDER BUYING THIS BOOK. IT COULD CHANGE YOUR LIFE!

The Vivos Splint and the DNA Splint to
expand the palate are different than the
one identified as a problem with the
AGGA appliance on CBS News investigation
See YouTube vivos.com
and holisticmouthsolutions.com
to understand the difference

Chapter 5

How the Meridian Chart
Reflects Fibromyalgia Symptoms

Faith is permitting ourselves to be sized by the thing we do not see.
~ Martin Luther

In the late 1940's, Dr Reinhard Voll, a German medical doctor, began researching traditional Chinese medicine. He confirmed that acupuncture points have distinct properties connected to surrounding tissue. He initially validated 850 points on the hands and feet that Chinese acupuncture used to correspond to organs, glands and tissue. He also verified that each tooth is connected to various organs, tissues and glands in the body via meridians, also referred to as the body's energy highway. We now recognize that we can find evidence of overall health and wellness by reviewing dental conditions. Numerous dental charts depicting the interrelationship between teeth and organs have been published, some of which can be explored at www.biologicalmedicineinstitue.com, or https://meridiantoothchart.com. These are interactive sites where readers can explore the connections between teeth and organs and investigate potential correspondences to consider with their primary care team.

As I mentioned in chapter 1, I went to see Dr Robert Dronyk, a naturopathic chiropractor in London, Ontario. When I discussed my fibromyalgia symptoms with him, I mentioned that they had started after the dental work that I had received. He showed me a meridian tooth chart on pages 74 and 75. As we examined the symptoms that I was experiencing, it was evident that many of my fibromyalgia symptoms seem to be directly related to the hitting of tooth 13, when I tapped my teeth together. This was exactly where the dental bridge was located. While the list below is not comprehensive, these were some of the issues that I was experiencing, and which corresponded to the hitting tooth 13, as per the meridian tooth chart on pages 74 and 75:

- Shoulder and neck pain, with an inability to turn my head to the left
- Shoulder rolled forward
- Soreness in my chest, rapid pulse
- Bruising
- Sciatica, low back pain
- Constipation, indigestion and bloating
- Left ankle seemed to twist easily
- Catch my L big toes when I walked
- Pain down left side
- Tendonitis
- Carpal tunnel
- Panic attacks
- Chills and sweating mostly at night
- Cold hands and feet
- Balance was off, running into walls

I had also been experiencing compromised airway symptoms stemming from my tongue blocking my airway. These symptoms included:

- Lack of concentration
- Dreams
- Difficulty sleeping
- Snoring
- Several sore throats
- Extreme fatigue

- Difficulty swallowing pills
- Biting the Left side of my cheek
- Tongue scalloped around edges

Additionally, after consulting Dr. Dronyk, I came to understand that the following symptoms were likely related to my temporomandibular joint dysfunction which caused muscle spasm in the muscles around my jaw.

- Black spots floating in front of my eyes
- Twitching in my Left eye
- Grinding my teeth
- Migraine headaches
- Muscle spasm in my jaw

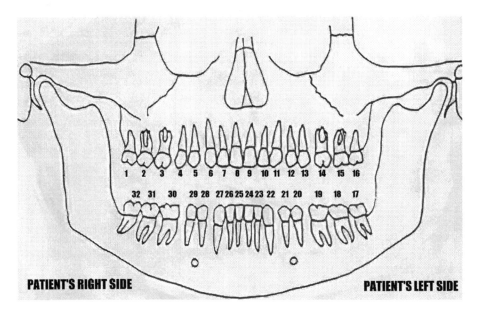

THE NUMBER GIVEN TO EACH TOOTH
Courtesy of Dr. Dawn Ewing
www.drdawn.net
Let the Tooth Be Known

Organs	Joints	Vertebrae	Endocrine	Systems	Sensory	Muscles	Sinus	Patient's Right Side
Heart Terminal Ileum Ileo-Cecal Area	Ulnar side of shoulder, Hand and Elbow Plantar side of Foot Toes Sacro-Iliac	C - 1, 2, 7 TH - 1, 5, 6, 7 S - 1, 2		Peripheral Nerves Energy Exchange	Middle Ext. Ear Tongue	Psoas		32
Lung, Large Intestine Ileo-Cecal Area	Radial side of Shoulder, Hand and Elbow Foot Big Toe	C - 1, 2, 5, 6, 7 TH - 2, 3, 4 L - 4, 5		Arteries (31) Veins (30)	Nose	Quadriceps (31) Gracilis (30) Sartorius (30)	Ethmoid	31 30
Esophagus Stomach Pancreas Pylorus Pyloric Antrum	Anterior Hip Anterior Knee Medial Ankle Jaw	C - 1, 2 TH - 11, 12 L - 1	Ovary and Testicle (28)	Lymph (29) Breast	Tongue	Pect Maj Sternal (29) Quadratus Lumborum (28) Hamstring	Maxillary	29 28
Liver Gallbladder Biliary Ducts	Posterior Knee Hip Lateral Ankle	C - 1, 2 TH - 8, 9, 10	Ovary Testicle		Anterior Eye	Gluteus Maximus	Sphenoid	27
Kidney Bladder Ovary/Testicle Prostate/Uterus Rectum/Anus	Posterior Knee Sacro-coccygeal Posterior ankle	C - 1, 2 L - 2, 3 S - 3, 4, 5 Coccyx	Adrenals			Tensor Fasciae Latae (26) Pyriformis (26) Gluteus Medius (25)	Frontal Sphenoid	26 25
Kidney Bladder Ovary/Testicle Prostate/Uterus Rectum/Anus	Posterior Knee Sacro-coccygeal Posterior ankle	C - 1, 2 L - 2, 3 S - 3, 4, 5 Coccyx	Adrenals			Tensor Fasciae Latae (23) Pyriformis (23) Gluteus Medius (24)	Frontal Sphenoid	24 23
Liver Biliary Ducts	Posterior Knee Hip Lateral Ankle	C - 1, 2 TH - 8, 9, 10	Ovary Testicle		Anterior Eye	Gluteus Maximus	Sphenoid	22
Esophagus Stomach Spleen	Anterior Hip Anterior Knee Medial Ankle Jaw	C - 1, 2 TH - 11, 12 L - 1	Ovary and Testicle (21)	Lymph (20) Breast	Tongue	Pect Maj Sternal (20) Quadratus Lumborum (21) Hamstring	Maxillary	21 20
Lung Large Intestine	Radial side of Shoulder, Hand and Elbow Foot Big Toe	C - 1, 2, 5, 6, 7 TH - 2, 3, 4 L - 4, 5		Arteries (18) Veins (19)	Nose	Quadriceps (18) Gracilis (19) Sartorius (19)	Ethmoid	19 18
Heart Ileum Jejunum	Ulnar side of shoulder, Hand and Elbow, Plantar side of Foot, Toes, Sacro-Iliac	C - 1, 2, 7 TH - 1, 5, 6, 7 S - 1, 2		Peripheral Nerves Energy Exchange	Middle Ext. Ear Tongue	Psoas		17

Dental Meridian Chart Copyright 2002 Courtesy of Dr. Dawn Ewing Holistic Alternatives www.drdawn.net

MERIDIAN TOOTH CHART - Description available on pages 82-92.

Patient's Right Side	Sinus	Muscles	Sensory	Systems	Endocrine	Vertebrae	Joints	Organs
1		Trapezius	Internal Ear Tongue	Central Nervous Limbic	Ant. Pituitary	C - 1, 2, 7 TH - 1, 5, 6, 7 S - 1, 2	Ulnar side of Shoulder, Hand and Elbow Plantar side of Foot, Toes, Sacro-Iliac	Heart Terminal Ileum Duodenum
2 / 3	Maxillary	Abdominal (2) Latissimus (3)	Oropharynx Larynx Tongue	Breast	Thyroid (3) Parathyroid (2)	C - 1, 2 TH - 11, 12 L - 1	Jaw, Ant. Hip Ant. Knee Medial Ankle	Pancreas Stomach Esophagus
4 / 5	Ethmoid	Diaphragm (4) Pectoralis Maj. Clavicular Coracobrachialis Popliteus (5)	Nose	Breast (4)	Thymus (4) Post. Pituitary (5)	C - 1, 2, 5, 6, 7 TH - 2, 3, 4 L - 4, 5	Radial side of Shoulder, Hand and Elbow Foot Big Toe	Lung Large Intestine Bronchi
6	Sphenoid	Deltoid Ant. Serratus	Posterior Eye		Intermediate Pituitary Hypothalamus	C - 1, 2 TH - 8, 9, 10	Posterior Knee Hip Lateral Ankle	Liver Gallbladder Biliary Ducts
7 / 8	Frontal Sphenoid	Subscapularis (7) Neck-Flex and Ext (8)	Nose		Pineal	C - 1, 2 L - 2, 3 S - 3, 4, 5 Coccyx	Posterior Knee Sacro-coccygeal Posterior Ankle	Kidney, Bladder Ovary/Testicle Prostate/Uterus Rectum/Anus
9 / 10	Frontal Sphenoid	Subscapularis(10) Neck-Flex and Ext (9)	Nose		Pineal	C - 1, 2 L - 2, 3 S - 3, 4, 5 Coccyx	Posterior Knee Sacro-coccygeal Posterior Ankle	Kidney, Bladder Ovary/Testicle Prostate/Uterus Rectum/Anus
11	Sphenoid	Deltoid Ant. Serratus	Posterior Eye		Intermediate Pituitary Hypothalamus	C - 1, 2 TH - 8, 9, 10	Posterior Knee Hip Lateral Ankle	Liver Biliary Ducts
12 / 13	Ethmoid	Diaphragm (13) Pectoralis Maj. Clavicular Coracobrachialis Popliteus (12)	Nose	Breast (13)	Thymus (13) Post. Pituitary (12)	C - 1, 2, 5, 6, 7 TH - 2, 3, 4 L - 4, 5	Radial side of Shoulder, Hand and Elbow Foot Big Toe	Lung Large Intestine Bronchi
14 / 15	Maxillary	Abdomial (15) Lattisimus (14)	Oropharynx Larynx Tongue	Breast	Thyroid (14) Parathyroid (15)	C - 1, 2 TH - 11, 12 L - 1	Jaw, Ant. Hip Ant. Knee Medial Ankle	Spleen Stomach Esophagus
16		Trapezius	Internal Ear Tongue	Central Nervous Limbic	Ant. Pituitary	C - 1, 2, 7 TH - 1, 5, 6, 7 S - 1, 2	Ulnar side of shoulder, Hand and Elbow, Plantar side of Foot, Toes, Sacro-Iliac	Heart Duodenum Jejunum Ileum

Dental Meridian Chart Copyright 2002 Courtesy of Dr. Dawn Ewing Holistic Alternatives www.drdawn.net

MERIDIAN TOOTH CHART - Description available on pages 82-92.

If we examine the tooth-organ meridian chart on page 75, tooth # 13 you will see the correspondence between my symptoms and the meridian:

- Ethmoid cells : is the lining of the sinuses, I had sinus problems
- Shoulder : I had shoulder pain
- Elbow : I had tendonitis of the elbow
- Hand radial side: that is the thumb side. I had carpal tunnel
- Foot and big toe: I would twist my left ankle easily and would catch my big toe when I walked
- C 5,5,7: the cervical spine in your neck. I could not turn my neck all the way to the left
- T 2,3,4,: the thoracic spine which affects the mid chest. I had soreness in my chest
- L 4,5: The lumbar spine which affects the lower back. I had sciatic and lower back pain
- Lung: I do not recall lung issues specifically
- Large intestines: I was constipated, and bloated which I contributed to not drinking enough water
- Thymus and posterior pituitary: I was unaware of symptoms
- Breast: I had thickening of my left breast and required repeat mammograms

I believe that tooth 13 seen on the chart was also the tooth I had the root canal on twice. This tooth was pulled when the bridge was removed, and my symptoms subsided. The correlation between the tooth issue, my physical symptoms, and the correspondences on the chart were significant

If you have difficulty reading this chart go to meridiantoothchart.com on the internet and you may be able to read it more clearly.

It is important that you look closely at the meridian tooth chart so that you will be able to assess yourself to determine how the meridians tooth chart affects you.

As I have continued to explore these correspondences, I discovered Dr Dawn Ewing. She was a dental hygienist that returned to school completing her doctorate thesis on the meridian-tooth connection. Her website www.drdawn.net will clarify the connection between the meridians, teeth, and other parts of the body. It is also a good source of information for other aspects of dental care. Her chart on pages 74 and 75 can be seen in colour and can be purchased on her website. Dr Dawn Ewing discussed meridians and how energy travels throughout our body. The meridians relate back to Chinese medicine and are the basis of acupuncture and reflexology. You can read about this in her book "Let the Tooth be Known". Which can be purchased through her website (www.dr.dawn.net) where there are very clear explanations of meridians by Dr. Reinhard Voll and Dr. Dawn Ewing.

Although a deeper understanding of the details of tooth-meridian correspondence is an interesting study, a detailed understanding may not be necessary when examining symptom-tooth correspondence. I use this chart when I interview fibromyalgia patients. I have the patient tap their teeth together and tell me which tooth that they notice hitting first. When we look at the meridian tooth chart and follow the column down that relates to that specific tooth, we often reveal symptom complaints in the entire body experienced by the patient. Having a chart that allows me to predict, and explain his or her symptoms, gives people hope, especially when the interview occurs over the phone.

Case Study:

Kelly was someone that I interviewed, who had been experiencing various symptoms. She complained of blurred vision, had been hospitalized for inflammation of the liver, gallbladder and common bile duct, pain in her hips and knees, and was experiencing heart palpitations. When we explored further, it was discovered that she was hitting her eye tooth first (tooth number 6 on the dental meridian chart).

I have also interviewed eight people with Sjogren's Syndrome. Two of their symptoms are dry eyes and dry mouth. All eight of them were hitting their front teeth first. I have found it difficult finding individuals with this syndrome so I do not know if this is consistent with everybody with this disease, however these findings are suggestive of a correlation.

I have also noticed that men that have prostate issues are frequently hitting their front teeth first. While I do not know if this is a cause and effect relationship, it is interesting to note that Dr Dawn Ewing does mention this in one of her podcasts.

Individuals who are experiencing fibromyalgia symptoms often are challenged with being unable to find any concrete answers to their concerns. My goal in using the meridian tooth chart is to support fibromyalgia patients to consider the possibility that their teeth may be part of the mystery behind their symptoms.

I was blessed when I was experiencing fibromyalgia, TMJ and airway symptoms that God directed me to all of the right professionals to alleviate my symptoms: I went to Dr Robert Dronyk a naturopathic chiropractor who gave me the meridian chart and explained the correspondence between my symptoms and the meridian of my teeth. I went to Dr Daniel Gole, a dentist in Hasting, Michigan who recognized that my dental bridge was placed incorrectly, removed it. Immediately my fibromyalgia symptoms disappeared. I went to Dr Brock Rondeau, a dentist in London, Ontario to have my bottom jaw brought forward 7mm with a double splint on my teeth which alleviated my migraines, and opened my airway. I had braces put on by Dr Rondeau for 1 1/2 years. This has realigned my teeth and bite. Without these amazing dentists who both belonged to The Head Neck and Facial Pain Dental Organization, I would still be in pain and have difficulty sleeping.

You cannot expect traditionally trained dentists to have this knowledge. I went to several of these dentists who were unable to identify my problem. No one had identified that I had TMJ, nor did they recognize that my bite was off, or that my dental bridge was not placed correctly. It is critical to be your own advocate, and to do research for information for yourself. Dentists do not learn this information in dental school. It is critical to find the correct information, and the right professionals who have chosen to take courses and expand their knowledge in order to help you.

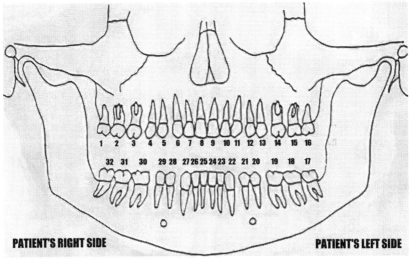

Courtesy of Dr. Dawn Ewing

In her book Let the Tooth be Known Dr. Dawn Ewing shares this above diagram to illustrate how dentists number each tooth in the mouth. In order to determine the correspondences, determine which tooth is hitting first, and verify the number of the tooth. Once the correspondence has been determined, an exploration of the accord between symptoms and tooth can be explored on the meridian tooth chart. An interactive tooth meridian chart, and corresponding explanations can be found at biologicalmedicine institute.com, where it is possible to explore the correlations between teeth, symptoms and meridians.

Normal adults have 32 teeth: 16 on each of the upper and lower jaw, which typically erupt by age 13. There are typically 4 incisors, or front teeth, 2 canines, which are next to the incisors, 4 premolars, and 6 molars which extend to the back of the mouth. According to traditional Chinese medicine, and acupuncture, there are 12 meridians, with a meridian related to each tooth, and which are the energy channels which pass through the body. It is this acupuncture meridian chart that illustrates why symptoms extend from teeth through the body.

You can find a coloured photo of the meridians on the web at <u>twelve meridian</u> <u>chart on the body,</u> as illustrated below. Each tooth correlates with one of these twelve meridians.

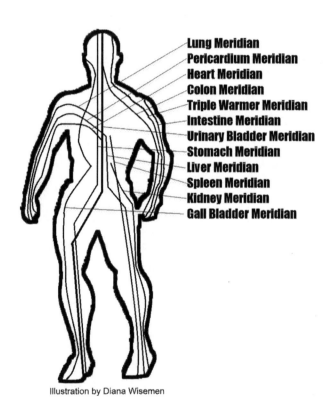

Lung Meridian
Pericardium Meridian
Heart Meridian
Colon Meridian
Triple Warmer Meridian
Intestine Meridian
Urinary Bladder Meridian
Stomach Meridian
Liver Meridian
Spleen Meridian
Kidney Meridian
Gall Bladder Meridian

Illustration by Diana Wisemen

I invite you to refer to Dr. Dawn Ewing's website for a more detailed description of the correspondences.

THE MERIDIAN TOOTH CHART EXPLANATION (see dental number) This information can be found on Dr Dawn Ewing's tooth chart @ drdawn.net as well as a slightly different version at meridiantoothchart.com.

For example: If one is hitting the right wisdom tooth first. It is Tooth #1

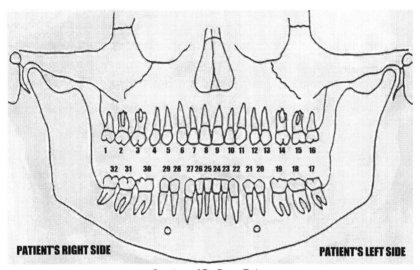

Courtesy of Dr. Dawn Ewing

THE NUMBER GIVEN TO EACH TOOTH
Courtesy of Dr. Dawn Ewing
www.drdawn.net
Let the Tooth Be Known

Look at the organs, glands, vertebrae, and sense organs etc on the meridian tooth chart #1 below and the intestine on the 12 meridian chart on page 80. Tap your teeth together, if you are hitting one tooth first, identify the number of the tooth looking at the tooth chart. The symptoms related to each tooth are as follows according to the meridian.

Refer to the dental chart on page 81 for the numbers of the teeth.
Some of the teeth share the same meridian: Teeth 2&3, 4&5, 7&8, 9&10, 12&13, 14&15, 18&19, 20&21, 23&24, 25&26, 28&29, 30&31 with minor differences.
Note: The dermatomes were not included for these teeth.

Tooth # 1 Upper Right Third Molar (wisdom tooth) Meridian

Organs: R side of the heart, R terminal ileum, duodenum
Endocrine: Anterior pituitary
Vertebrae: Cervical 1,2,7; Thoracic 1,5,6,7; Sacral 1,2
Sensory: R inner ear, tongue on R side
Systems: Central nervous and limbic
Muscular: Trapezius
Joint: Ulnar side of R shoulder, R hand and R elbow, R plantar side of R foot, R toes, sacral-iliac on R
Sinus: None

Tooth # 2 Upper Right Second Molar Meridian

Organs: Pancreas, R side of stomach, esophagus
Endocrine: R side parathyroid
Vertebrae: Cervical 1,2; Thoracic 11,12; Lumbar 1
Sensory: Oropharynx, larynx, tongue R side
Systems: R breast
Muscles: R side abdominal muscle
Joints: R jaw, right anterior hip, R anterior knee, R medial ankle
Sinus: Maxillary

Tooth # 3 Upper Right First Molar Meridian

Organs: Pancreas, R side of stomach, esophagus
Endocrine: R side of thyroid
Vertebrae: Cervical 1,2; Thoracic 11,12; Lumbar 1
Sensory: Oropharynx, larynx, R side tongue
Systems: R breast
Muscles: R side latissimus dorsi
Joints: R jaw, R anterior hip, R anterior knee, R medial ankle
Sinus: Maxillary

Tooth # 4 Upper Right Second Bicuspid Meridian

Organs: R lung, large intestine on R side, R bronchi
Endocrine: Thymus
Vertebrae: Cervical 1,2,5,6,7; Thoracic 2,3,4; Lumbar 4,5
Sensory: R side of nose
Systems: R breast
Muscles: R side of diaphragm, R pectoralis major clavicular
Joints: R radial side of shoulder, hand and elbow; R foot, R big toe
Sinus: Ethmoid

Tooth # 5 Upper Right Second First Bicuspid Meridian

Organs: R lung, large intestine on R side, R bronchi
Endocrine: Posterior lobe of pituitary
Vertebrae: Cervical 1,2,5,6,7; Thoracic 2,3,4; Lumbar 4,5
Sensory: R side of nose
Systems: None
Muscles: R pectoralis major clavicular, R coracobrachialis popliteus
Joints: R radial side of shoulder, R hand and R elbow; R foot, R big toe
Sinus: Ethmoid

Tooth # 6 Upper Right Cuspid Meridian

Organs: R side of liver, gallbladder, biliary ducts on right side
Endocrine: Intermediate lobe of pituitary, hypothalamus
Vertebrae: Cervical 1,2; Thoracic 8,9,10
Sensory: R posterior eye
System: None
Muscles: R deltoid, R anterior serratus
Joints: R posterior knee, R hip, R lateral ankle
Sinus: Sphenoid and tonsilla palate

Tooth # 7 Upper Right Lateral Incisor Meridian

Organs: R kidneys, R side of bladder, R ovary/testicle, prostate/uterus, rectum/anus
Endocrine: Pineal gland
Vertebrae: Cervical 1,2; Lumbar 2,3; Sacral 3,4,5; Coccyx
Sensory: Nose
Systems: None
Muscles: R subscapularis
Joints: R posterior knee, R sacro-coccygeal, R posterior ankle
Sinus: R frontal & sphenoid

Tooth # 8 Upper Right Central Incisor (R Front Tooth) Meridian

Organs: R kidney, right side of bladder, R ovary/testicle, prostate/uterus, rectum/anus
Endocrine: Pineal gland
Vertebrae: Cervical 1,2; Lumbar 2,3; Sacral 3,4,5; Coccyx
Sensory: Nose
Systems: None
Muscles: R neck-flexors and extensors
Joints: R Posterior knee, R sacro-coccygeal, R posterior ankle
Sinus: R frontal & sphenoid

Tooth # 9 Upper Left Central Incisor (L Front Tooth) Meridian

Organs: L kidney bladder, L ovary/testicle, prostate/uterus, rectum/anus
Endocrine: Pineal gland
Vertebrae: Cervical 1,2; Lumbar 2,3; Sacral 3,4,5; Coccyx
Sensory: Nose
Systems: None
Muscles: L neck-flexor and extensors
Joints: L posterior knee, L sacra-coccygeal, L posterior ankle
Sinus: L frontal & L sphenoid

Tooth # 10 Upper Left Lateral Incisor Meridian

Organs: L kidney, bladder, L ovary/testicle, prostate/uterus, rectum/anus
Endocrine: Pineal gland
Vertebrae: Cervical 1,2; Lumbar 2,3; Sacral 3,4,5; Coccyx
Sensory: Nose
Systems: None
Muscles: L subscapularis
Joints: L posterior knee, L sacra-coccygeal, L posterior ankle
Sinus: L frontal & L sphenoid

Tooth # 11 Upper Left Cuspid Meridian

Organs: L side of liver, L side of bile duct
Endocrine: Intermediate lobe of pituitary gland, hypothalamus
Vertebrae: Cervical 1,2; Thoracic 8,9,10
Sensory: L posterior eye
Systems: None
Muscles: L deltoid, L anterior serratus
Joints: L posterior knee, L hip, L lateral ankle
Sinus: L sphenoid & tonsilla palate

Tooth # 12 Upper Left First Meridian

Organs: L lung, large intestine on the left, L bronchi
Endocrine: posterior lobe of pituitary gland
Vertebrae: Cervical 1,2,5,6,7; Thoracic 2,3,4; Lumbar 4,5
Sensory: L side of nose
Systems: None
Muscles: Pectoralis major clavicular, L coracobrachialis popliteus
Joints: radial side of left shoulder, L hand, and L elbow; L foot, L big toe
Sinus: Ethmoid

Tooth # 13 Upper Left Second Bicuspid Meridian

Organs: L lung, large intestine on the left, L bronchi
Endocrine: thymus
Vertebrae: Cervical 1,2,5,6,7; Thoracic 2,3,4; Lumbar 4,5
Sensory: Left side of nose
Systems: L breast
Muscles: L diaphragm, L pectoralis major clavicular
Joints: Radial side of left shoulder, L hand, L elbow, L foot and
L big toe
Sinus: Ethmoid

Tooth # 14 Upper Left First Molar Meridian

Organs: Spleen, stomach left side, esophagus
Endocrine: Thyroid
Vertebrae: Cervical 1,2; Thoracic 11,12; Lumbar 1
Sensory: Oropharynx, larynx, tongue on left
Systems: L breast
Muscles: L latissimus dorsi
Joints: L jaw, anterior L hip, anterior L knee, L medial ankle
Sinus: Maxillary

Tooth # 15 Upper Left Second Molar Meridian

Organs: Spleen, stomach left side, esophagus
Endocrine: Parathyroid gland
Vertebrae: Cervical 1,2; Thoracic 11,12; Lumbar 1
Sensory: Oropharynx, larynx, tongue on left
Systems: L breast
Muscles: L abdominal muscle
Joints: L jaw, anterior L hip, L anterior knee, L medial ankle
Sinus: Maxillary

Tooth # 16 Upper Left Third Molar (wisdom tooth) Meridian

Organs: L side of heart, duodenum, jejunum, ileum
Endocrine: Anterior lobe of pituitary gland
Vertebrae: Cervical 1,2,7; Thoracic 1,5,6,7; Sacral 1,2
Sensory: L internal ear, L side of tongue
Systems: Central nervous and limbic
Muscles: Mid trapezius
Joints: Ulnar side of L shoulder, L hand, L elbow; plantar side of L foot and toes; L side of sacral-iliac joint
Sinus: None

BOTTOM TEETH LEFT TO RIGHT

Tooth # 17 Third Molar (wisdom) Meridian

Organs: L side of heart, ileum, jejunum
Endocrine: None
Vertebrae: Cervical 1,2,7; Thoracic 1,5,6,7; Sacral 1,2
Sensory: Middle ext. ear and tongue
Systems: Peripheral nerves energy exchange
Muscles: Psoas
Joints: Ulnar side of left shoulder, L hand and L elbow; plantar side of L foot

and toes; L sacral-iliac joint
Sinus: None

Tooth # 18 Lower Left Second Molar Meridian

Organs: L side of large intestine, L lung
Endocrine: None
Vertebrae: Cervical 1,2,5,6,7; Thoracic 2,3,4; Lumbar 4,5
Sensory: Nose
Systems: Arteries
Muscles: L quadriceps
Joints: Radial side of L shoulder, L hand, L elbow, L foot and L big toe
Sinus: Ethmoid

Tooth # 19 Lower Left First Molar Meridian

Organs: L side of large intestine, L lung
Endocrine: None
Vertebrae: Cervical 1,2 5,6,7; Thoracic 2,3,4; Lumbar 4,5
Sensory: Nose
Systems: Veins
Muscles: L muscle gracilis and sartorius
Joints: Radial side of L shoulder, L hand, L elbow, L foot and L big toe
Sinus: Ethmoid

Tooth # 20 Lower Left Second Bicuspid Meridian

Organs: Esophagus, stomach on L side, spleen
Endocrine: L mammary glands
Vertebrae: Cervical 1,2; Thoracic 11,12; Lumbar 1
Sensory: Tongue
Systems: Lymph and L breast

Muscles: L pectorals major, sternal, hamstrings
Joints: Anterior L hip, anterior L knee, L medial ankle, L jaw
Sinus: L maxillary

Tooth # 21 Lower Left First Bicuspid Meridian

Organs: Esophagus, stomach on L side, spleen
Endocrine: L mammary glands and L gonads
Vertebrae: Cervical 1,2; Thoracic 11,12; Lumbar 1
Sensory: Tongue
Systems: L breast, L gonads
Muscles: L quadratus lumborum, hamstrings
Joints: Anterior L hip, anterior L knee, medial L ankle, L jaw
Sinus: L maxillary

Tooth # 22 Lower Left Cuspid Meridian

Organs: L side of liver, L biliary ducts
Endocrine: L ovary, L testicle
Vertebrae: Cervical 1,2; Thoracic 8,9,10
Sensory: L anterior eye
Systems: None
Muscles: Gluteus maximus
Joints: L posterior knee, L hip, L lateral ankle
Sinus: Sphenoid

Tooth # 23 Lower Left Lateral Incisor Meridian

Organs: Left kidney, bladder, L ovary/testicle, prostate/uterus, rectum/anus
Endocrine: Adrenals
Vertebrae: Cervical 1,2; Lumbar 2,3; Sacral 3,4,5; Coccyx
Sensory: None
Systems: None
Muscles: L tensor fasciae latae, L pyroformis

Joints: L posterior knee, L sacra-coccygeal, posterior L ankle
Sinus: Frontal and sphenoid

Tooth # 24 Lower Left Central Incisor Meridian

Organs: L kidney, bladder, L ovary/testicle, prostate/uterus, rectum/anus
Endocrine: Adrenals
Vertebrae: Cervical 1,2; Lumbar 2,3; Sacral 3,4,5; Coccyx
Sensory: None
Systems: None
Muscles: Gluteus medius on the L side
Joints: L posterior knee, L sacro-coccygeal, L posterior ankle
Sinus: Frontal and sphenoid

Tooth # 25 Lower Right Central Incisor Meridian

Organs: R kidney bladder, R ovary/testicle, prostate/uterus, rectum/anus
Endocrine: Adrenals
Vertebrae: Cervical 1,2; Lumbar 2,3; Sacral 3,4,5; Coccyx
Sensory: None
Systems: None
Muscles: Gluteus medius on the R side
Joints: R posterior knee, R sacro-coccygeal, posterior R ankle
Sinus: Frontal and sphenoid

Tooth # 26 Lower Right Lateral Incisor Meridian

Organs: R kidney bladder, R ovary/testicle, prostate/uterus, rectum/anus
Endocrine: Adrenals
Vertebrae: Cervical 1,2; Lumbar 2,3; Sacral 3,4,5; Coccyx
Sensory: None
Systems: None
Muscles: R tensor fasciae latae, R pyroformis
Joints: R posterior knee, R sacro-coccygeal posterior R ankle

Sinus: Frontal and sphenoid

Tooth # 27 Lower Right Cuspid Meridian

Organs: R side of liver, gallbladder, biliary ducts right side
Endocrine: R ovary, R testicle
Vertebrae: Cervical 1,2; Thoracic 8,9,10
Sensory: Anterior R eye
Systems: None
Muscles: R gluteus maximus
Joints: R posterior knee, R hip, R lateral ankle
Sinus: Sphenoid

Tooth # 28 Lower Right First Bicuspid Meridian

Organs: Esophagus, right side of stomach, pancreas, R
Endocrine: R mammary glands, R gonads
Vertebrae: Cervical 1,2; Thoracic 11,12; Lumbar 1
Sensory: Tongue
Systems: Breast
Muscles: R quadratus lumborum, hamstrings
Joints: Anterior R hip, anterior R knee, R medial ankle and R jaw
Sinus: R maxillary

Tooth # 29 Lower Right Second Bicuspid Meridian

Organs: Esophagus, right side of stomach, pancreas, pylorus, pyloric antrum
Endocrine: R mammary glands
Vertebrae: Cervical 1,2; Thoracic 11,12; Lumbar 1
Sensory: Tongue
Systems: Lymph
Muscles: R pectoral major, sternal, hamstrings
Joints: Anterior R hip, anterior R knee, R medial ankle, R jaw
Sinus: R maxillary

Tooth # 30 Lower Right First Molar Meridian

Organs: R Lung, large intestine on right, ileo-cecal area
Endocrine: None
Vertebrae: Cervical 1,2,5,6,7; Thoracic 2,3,4; Lumbar 4,5
Sensory: Nose
Systems: Veins
Muscles: R muscle gracilis, sartorius
Joints: R radial side of shoulder, R hand and R elbow; R foot, R big toe
Sinus: Ethmoid

Tooth # 31 Lower R Second Molar Meridian

Organs: R lung, large intestine on R side, ileo-cecal area
Endocrine: None
Vertebrae: Cervical 1,2,5,6,7; Thoracic 2,3,4; Lumbar 4,5
Sensory: Nose
Systems: Arteries
Muscles: R quadriceps
Joints: R radial side of shoulder, R hand and R elbow; R foot, R big toe
Sinus: Ethmoid

Tooth # 32 Lower Right Third Molar (Wisdom tooth) Meridian

Organs: R side of heart, terminal ileum
Endocrine: None
Vertebrae: Cervical 1,2,7; Thoracic 1,5,6,7; Sacral 1,2
Sensory: Middle exterior ear, tongue
Systems: Peripheral nerves energy exchange
Muscles: Psoas
Joints: R ulnar side of shoulder, R hand and R elbow; plantar side of R foot and toes; sacro-iliac joint on right side
Sinus: None

This information can be found in Dr. Dawn Ewing book, "Let The Tooth Be Known" on pages 115-121, in greater depth to include the dermatomes. If you go to her website, www.drdawn.net, under Store tab, you can purchase the chart and her book.

Another chart can be found on meridiantoothchart.com, each tooth on the chart can be clicked on to see the organ meridian connection. There are several meridian tooth charts on the internet.

I know this information may be a little foreign to you. I am a nurse and had no knowledge about meridian until I thought my symptoms started with the placement of my dental bridge. Without Dr Dronyk, a naturopathic chiropractor's knowledge of meridians I may not have found the solution to my fibromyalgia.

For more explanation on meridians go to the You tube video " Healthy Living - A Conversation on Mouth/Body Health" with Dr Dawn Ewing.

Chapter 6

Case Studies

We cannot solve our problems with the same thinking
we used when we created them.
~ Albert Einstein

In this and the following chapter, I will be presenting case studies of individuals that I interviewed who have been suffering from fibromyalgia. If the reader does a detailed survey of these cases, they will notice that there all of these patients have TMJ symptoms, and all of these clients also have airway issues-either a narrow palate or evidence of the bottom jaw being too far back, which means that the tongue is too far back, and all have symptoms down the corresponding meridian. The following three case studies highlight clients who have a specific cluster of TMJ/ fibromyalgia symptoms related to a narrow palate, in addition to other dental issues. Chapter 7 will continue with additional case studies with individuals who had other, similar symptom resolution.

Case Study # 1:

Kelly is my daughter, a 48-year-old female who had at least 30 of the fibromyalgia symptoms. She had braces at age 10, and started having daily headaches, and migraines at age 12. Her everyday headaches went away when she was 21 years old. She had gone to a TMJ dentist and he removed the wire that the orthodontist had placed behind her two front teeth, after her braces were removed at age 12.

The TMJ dentist stated that the wire could not be placed across the midline of the two front teeth without affecting the nervous system. At 21, Kelly also had her palate expanded, and had braces reapplied. She related that she felt physically better. It was noted that Kelly was congenitally missing her lateral teeth and had 6 baby teeth still in her mouth since there were no adult teeth to push baby teeth out. An abnormality inherited from her grandmother. This problem left her with a small mouth. Her braces had pulled her teeth together, so no spaces were visible. It was not until she had a fall in 2020, at age 46 when she hit her head on the cement that her TMJ symptoms reoccurred. Kelly was hitting **tooth # 6 (**her eye tooth) when I assessed her. She had the symptoms down the meridian of the tooth that hit first. She was experiencing blurred vision, pain in her right hip, and had been hospitalized for inflammation in her gallbladder, liver and common bile duct.

Below are the symptoms that are identified on this meridian. Note: At the time the case studies in this chapter were done, a slightly different meridian tooth chart was used, which is not as extensive as Dr Dawn Ewing's meridian tooth chart.

Tooth # 6 Canine, Gallbladder and Liver Meridian
Organs: Heart, liver gallbladder
Glands: Pituitary posterior lobe
Spine: Thoracic 8,9,10
Sense organ: Eye
Musculature: Trunk musculature
Joints: Foot, hip, posterior knee

Kelly reported many TMJ symptoms when she filled out the TMJ questionnaire, and also exhibited symptoms of a compromised airway. She also had **psoriatic arthritis and was on Ortezla at a cost of $3400/month.** These symptoms were discussed in the sleep chapter. She is presently being treated by a TMJ dentist to alleviate her TMJ symptoms, balance her bite, so tooth # 6 does not hit first. Additionally, the TMJ dentist is also addressing her airway issues.

The splint that the TMJ dentist made her has brought her bottom jaw forward to alleviate her overbite and open up her airway. The splint has also worked well to decrease the spasm in her jaw muscles. Once Kelly's airway was opened, her psoriasis and psoriatic arthritis went away and she has stopped taking Ortezla. The oral splint that she wears on her bottom teeth has allowed her to sleep better and she has become a much happier and healthier person. The statement she made after getting her splint was. "Oh, my God, I can breathe again."

Medication:
Kelly had been taking Ortezla for psoriasis, and 2400mg of ibuprofen every day for years for her headaches. She has recently been told that she needed to stop taking the ibuprofen, as it was beginning to affect her liver enzymes. She was also taking multivitamins, and trazadone to sleep. Kelly no longer takes Otezla, nor ibuprofen.

Case Study # 2 DeDe:

DeDe Is a 69-year-old female who was diagnosed with fibromyalgia in her late 30s. She stated that as a child she had two teeth pulled because her teeth were crowded. This caused a significantly narrow palate when she was young and had braces. I measured her palate using a cotton roll that should fit across the upper palate. I could only fit about 3/4 of the roll across her palate. This indicated that her palate was too narrow. She reported that she always felt that her tongue did not fit in her mouth correctly. Clinically, it should be noted that she was missing 2 molars each on both her upper and lower jaws.

When the TMJ questionnaire was completed it was obvious that she had a TMJ dysfunction. On the next page, see the results of her TMJ questionnaire.

TMJ Symptoms:

- Do you get headaches? Yes
- Do you get migraine headaches? Yes
- Do you frequently have neck aches? Yes
- Or stiff neck muscles? Yes
- Have you ever had chronic shoulder pain? Yes
- Or back pain? No
- Are your teeth sore when you wake up? Yes
- Have your wisdom teeth been extracted? Yes
- Do you get headaches on the front and back of the head? Yes
- Have you ever had a severe blow to the head? Yes
- Any whiplash neck injuries? Yes, twice
- Are they any food you avoid eating? Yes
- Do you ever get dizzy? Yes
- Do you ever feel faint? Yes
- Do you ever feel nauseated? Yes
- Do you hear ringing, buzzing, or hissing sounds in either ear? Yes
- Do you have allergies? Yes
- Do you have sinus problems? Yes
- Do you snore at night? Yes
- Have you ever been involved in a serious accident ? Yes
- Do you feel or hear a clicking popping or cracking noise in your jaw? Yes
- Has your jaw ever locked when you were unable to open or close? Yes
- Do you wear glasses? Yes
- Are there times when your eyesight blurs? Yes
- Do you get pain in, around or behind either eye? Yes
- Is your nose stuffy when you do not have a cold? Yes
- Have you been diagnosed with Sleep Apnea? Yes
- Have you had a sleep study done at a Sleep Clinic? Yes

I used a more extensive fibromyalgia questionnaire when I assessed DeDe in order to get a more complete picture of her symptoms.

Note: She had several teeth pulled when she had braces when she was younger, causing a narrow palate.

DeDe's Fibromyalgia Symptoms:

- Attract mosquitoes and black flies
- Fatigue
- Crave carbohydrates
- Frequent yeast infections
- Overgrowing connective tissue, nail ridges
- Wide body aches and pains
- Have sleep apnea
- Experience frequent frustration
- Night sweats
- Delayed reaction until the next day if too active physically
- Get the shakes when you are hungry
- Bruise easily
- Recent fluorescent light bother you
- Have electromagnetic sensitivity /affected by storms
- Has numbness and tingling in feet and legs
- Has had serious illnesses / pulmonary embolus
- Unusual degree of clumsiness
- Sinus stuffiness
- Frequent runny nose
- Trouble swallowing
- Ear pain occasionally
- Fluctuating blood pressure
- Dry eyes, and mouth all the time
- Problem swallowing and chewing
- Red or tearing eyes
- Popping or clicking of the jaw
- Itchy ears
- Unexplained toothache
- Eye pain

- Blurry vision
- Dizziness when you turn your head
- Pain mid-shoulder when carrying heavy purse
- Pain when you writes, a changing signature, illegible handwriting
- Esophageal reflux
- Chest tightness
- Hiatus hernia
- Intestinal cramps, bloating
- Nausea
- Irritable bladder or bowel
- Pain with intercourse
- Menstrual problems
- Low back pain, sciatica
- Shin splints
- Stumble over her own feet
- Lower leg cramps
- Foot pain
- Numbness or hypersensitivity R leg
- First walk in morning like walking on nails

After doing all of these extensive questionnaires, I came to believe that DeDe's fibromyalgia symptoms were related to her TMJ, her compromised airway further, corresponded to symptoms down the meridian of the teeth that hit first.

Airway symptoms below are as outlined by Dr James Garry's (Dentist) questionnaire:

DeDe's Airway Symptoms:

- Frequent night-time awakening
- Stomach acid reflux and heartburn
- Snoring
- Disturbing dreams

- Chest wall soreness
- Morning headaches
- Frequent nausea
- Gag easily on food or pills
- Unexplained weight gain
- Grogginess and dizziness
- Dry lips
- Headaches in the frontal, and occipital lobe
- High narrow palate
- Chewing cheek
- Constantly tired
- Bloodshot eyes
- Chronic ear aches as a child
- Chronic throat infections
- Severe fatigue
- Constantly tired

I concluded that DeDe had all of these airway symptoms due to her narrow palate. She further related that her tongue does not seem to fit in her mouth properly. A CAT scan of her airway was performed at the Breath Well Sleep Well Clinic, which showed that DeDe had a compromised airway www.breathewellsleepwellclearwater.com. It was further noted in her medical records that she had severe sleep apnea and it was confirmed that she was diagnosed with a narrow upper palate.

In addition to the above noted assessments, DeDe was assessed using the meridian chart. DeDe felt she was hitting two teeth first: tooth 5 and tooth 10. She was exhibiting symptoms down the meridian of each of those teeth.

Tooth # 5 First Premolar, Large intestine meridian

Organs: Stomach, pancreas, liver, large intestine, right lung
Glands: Pituitary posterior lobe, thyroid
Spine: Cervical 5,6,7; Thoracic 3,4; Lumbar 4,5

Sense organs: ethmoid cells (lining of sinus) eye maxillary sinus
Musculature: trunk and extremities musculature
Joints: radial hand, foot, big toe, shoulder, elbow

Tooth # 10 Left Second Incisor, Bladder Meridian

Organs: Left kidney, bladder, urogenital
Glands: Pineal
Spine: Lumbar 2,3; Sacral 3,4,5; Coccyx
Sense organ: Frontal sinus
Musculature: Lower extremities
Joints: Foot, sacrum & coccyx

When DeDe's fibromyalgia symptoms are examined, one can see how the symptoms relate to the meridians. DeDe had an extensive history of internal medical concerns: she experienced kidney stones, bladder suspension, hysterectomy, deviated septum and sinus surgery. Additionally, she had her gallbladder and appendix removed, a history of bilateral blood clots in her lungs. She had a right knee replacement, and she further experienced chest pain and stomach pain. She had polyps removed during a colonoscopy, and was also experiencing sleep apnea, and pain in her right leg.

Treatment:

DeDe went to the Breath Well Sleep Well Clinic in Clearwater, Florida and had a CAT Scan of her airway. With this diagnostic tool, she was shown to have severe sleep apnea with a narrow upper palate. Dr Rodeghero (dentist) in Clearwater fitted her with a "Vivos splint" to expand her narrow palate. I would refer the reader to vivos.com or YouTube to see the amazing results other patients have experienced from wearing the Vivos splint over a period of a year. Cathy at the Breathwell Sleepwell Clinic educated DeDe and her husband concerning how the mouth develops and how narrow palate affects the airway. They were also shown the CAT scan of her narrow airway and the treatment plan for using the Vivos splint to expand her airway.

If the reader will recall, DeDe had teeth removed when she had braces as a child. This is a childhood treatment which contributed to her narrow palate as an adult. At time of printing, DeDe has received a dental splint, and is adjusting the screw on her splint every two weeks with the goal to widen her palate and open up her airway.

Case Study # 3: Mya did not sleep well and had learning difficulties, not fibromyalgia but has a narrow palate.

I met Mya at my son's house and immediately noticed that she presented with a narrow smile. In the photos below, it can be noted that there were only four front teeth evident when she smiled. I had a conversation with her aunt, and asked if Mya had learning difficulties. I also suggested that the child likely did not sleep well, because of snoring, and that she had a narrow palate. Her aunt was surprised that I could tell just by looking at Mya that she snored, and that she had a high upper palate in her mouth. Mya also had large tonsils which made her a mouth breather. Mouth breathers often develop a high upper palate.

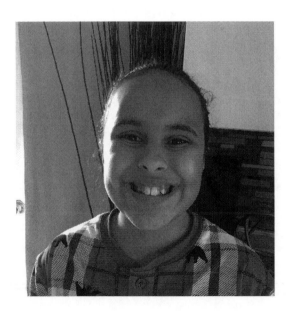

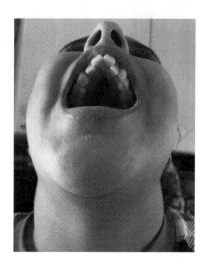

Since this initial encounter Mya was referred to a TMJ dentist. Mya has had her tonsils removed and is now in the process of getting her palate expanded by Dr Brock Rondeau a TMJ dentist in London, Ontario. Mya's grandmother cannot thank me enough for getting Mya the help that she needed to improve her airway and her dental health. Readers can support others within their sphere simply by recognizing an unusually narrow smile and suggesting that the individual be assessed by a good orthodontist.

Below is a photo of another girl before and after her palate was expanded.

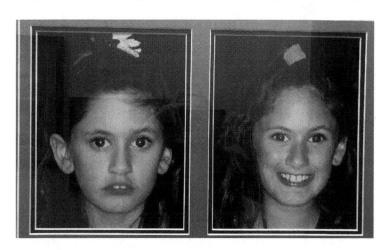

I invite the reader to go to Dr Ben Miraglia's youtube video, Connecting Sleep Disorder, where he discusses the link between ADHD and sleep deprivation. Mya had a narrow palate and enlarged tonsils, and could not sleep well because of impaired breathing at night. This may explain why she had difficulty learning, and why, when her palate is expanded, her sleep and her learning difficulties are expected to improve

Chapter 7 will discuss further case studies linking dental irregularities, TMJ and fibromyalgia disorders. I invite the reader to examine the case studies, and consider how they may relate to any symptoms that may be explained by these oral discrepancies.

Chapter 7

More Case Studies

We can't solve modern problems by going back in time.
Retreating to the safety of the familiar is an understandable response,
but God has called us to a life of faith. And faith requires us to face the
unknown while trusting Him completely.
~ Charles R. Swindoll

Case Study 1a: Jody:

Jody is a 48-year-old woman, who has been suffering with various symptoms since Sept of 1991. Jody's primary complaint of over thirty years, has been headaches. She was diagnosed with fibromyalgia. On the next page is the TMJ questionnaire that I used to assess possible TMJ involvement as related to client concerns.

TMJ HEALTH QUESTIONNAIRE

Name _____   Date _____

CHIEF CONCERN   Headaches

DATE OF ONSET   30 Years Ago

PAIN SYMPTOMS

Do you get headaches?	**Y** N	
Do you get migraine headaches?	Y **N**	
Do you frequently have neck aches or stiff neck muscles?	**Y** N	
Have you ever had chronic shoulder or back pain?	**Y** N	
Do you have trouble sleeping soundly?	**Y** N	
Are your jaws tired when you awaken?	**Y** N	
Are your teeth sore when you awaken?	**Y** N	
Have your wisdom teeth been extracted?	**Y** N	

Do you get headaches in the (right) or left temple areas? **Y** N

Do you get headaches in the (front) or back of your head? **Y** N

Do you clench your teeth during the day? **Y** N
Do you clench your teeth at night? **Y** N
Do you grind your teeth when asleep? **Y** N

When are your pain symptoms the worst?

Throughout the day

Does anything make you feel better?

No

What medications, if any, are you taking?
_____

How often do you take medication for relief of pain?
Never

TRAUMA OR ACCIDENTS

Have you ever had a severe blow to the head or jaw? **Y** N
Any whiplash neck injuries? Y **N**

Have you ever been involved in any serious accidents, such as a car accident? **Y** N
Details Hit by a car at age 6, knocked out a molar. Car accident age 16 -> loosened

JAW JOINT SYMPTOMS

Does your jaw feel tired after a big meal? Y **N**
Are there any foods you avoid eating? Y **N**
Do you ever get dizzy? **Y** N
Do you ever feel faint? **Y** N
Do you ever feel nauseated? **Y** N
Is there a family history of jaw joint (TMJ) problems or headaches? Y **N**

Do you feel or hear a 'clicking', 'popping' or 'cracking' noise from either jaw joint? **Y** N
Has your jaw ever locked when you were unable to open or close? **Y** N
Do you have difficulty opening wide or yawning? **Y** N
Have you ever had pain in either jaw joint? **Y** N
Does your jaw ache when you open wide? **Y** N

EAR AND EYE SYMPTOMS

Do you have pain in either ear? R **Y** N
Do you suffer from any loss of hearing? R **Y** N
Do you have itchiness or stuffiness in either ear? R **Y** N
Do you hear ringing, buzzing, or hissing sounds in either ear? Y **N**

Do you wear glasses or contacts? **Y** N
Are there times when your eyesight blurs? **Y** N
Do you get pain in, around or behind either eye? **Y** N

BREATHING

Do you have allergies? **Y** N
Do you have sinus problems? **Y** N
Do you snore at night? Y **N**

Is your nose stuffed when you don't have a cold? Y **N**
Have you been diagnosed with Sleep Apnea? Y **N**
Have you had a sleep study done at a Sleep Clinic (hospital)? Y **N**

Rev.03/20/09

Courtesy of Dr. Brock Rondeau

In addition to the symptoms described in the form on page 108, this client also has four front teeth that are on steel pegs.

Fibromyalgia Symptoms:

Jody experienced consistent shoulder and neck pain, and was unable to turn head to the right. She suffered a significant loss of concentration, and often had difficulty finding the right words when speaking. She reported feeling a "fullness" and itching in her ear. She related that she was always extremely tired. Jody often experienced chills and sweats most nights. She often experienced blurred vision in both eyes. She suffered from frequent panic attacks, soreness in her chest, and rapid pulse. Jody also had a lot of allergies, experienced sciatica and a lot of pain down the right side of her body. She noticed that her balance was off, that she was often running into the wall, and catching her right big toes when she walked. In addition to all of the above symptoms, she also experienced abdominal pain, back of neck pain, ear pain, frontal headaches and temporal headaches. She noticed that she was grinding her teeth, that she was experiencing temple and eyebrow pain, and significant temporomandibular joint pain.

Airway:

I was not measuring the upper palate or doing airway assessment at the time that I assessed Jody.

Meridian questionnaire:

Jody was hitting Tooth # 5

Tooth # 5 First Premolar, Large Intestine Meridian

Organs: Lung, large intestine, bronchi
Endocrine: Posterior pituitary

Vertebrae: Cervical 1,2,5,6,7; Thoracic 1,3,4; Lumbar 4,5
Sense organs: Ethmoid cells (lining of sinus)
Systems: Breast
Muscles: Diaphragm, pectoralis major, clavicular coracobrachialis, popliteus
Joints: Radial side of (shoulder, hand and elbow), R foot, R big toe
Sinus: Ethmoid

Jody's symptoms correlated with the meridian of Tooth # 5. She had difficulty turning her head, which corresponds to the cervical spine. She also experienced chest discomfort corresponding to the thoracic connection. Jody suffered from sciatica which is lumbar 4,5, and had pain down the right side of her body, and she consistently caught her big toe when she walked. Jody is planning on getting an appointment soon with the TMJ dentist, but unable to presently due to busyness at work.

Case# 2a: Meagan

History given by Meagan:

Meagan related that she had her wisdom teeth removed in 2006. She was unsure if her jaw was clicking prior to that procedure. She experienced a head injury at seven years old, which resulted in a concussion. In 2017 Meagan was diagnosed with adrenal fatigue. She has been having some mobility concerns, relating that she had difficulty navigating stairs, and walking. She was noticing a clicking in her left hip, and had received both an MRI and Xray of her left hip. They both showed a negative result. She was experiencing stiffness and pain in the right hip, and in her left knee. Meagan had significant black circles under her eyes. She had some significant neck restrictions when turning her head. Meagan stated that her left elbow was "loose". She was also on medication for acne. She stated that she was taking Botox shots in her neck and jaw to relieve neck spasms. She was receiving this treatment from a dentist. This treatment does relieve the pain, but the relief only lasts 3-4 months. This treatment is very expensive, with a cost of $1100 or more.

Megan's Fibromyalgia Symptoms:

Meagan has experienced a wide range of fibromyalgia which include restless leg syndrome, itchiness on the left leg, and the feeling of ants crawling under the skin of her left leg. She experienced extreme fatigue, she seemed to be highly attracted by mosquitoes and black flies. She realized that she was craving carbohydrates. She experienced generalized itching. She noticed that she was experiencing frequent frustration. Meagan had frequent yeast infections in her mouth, and that she has patches of skin with a painful network of fine veins and capillaries in her legs, that she was bruising easily. Meagan recognized that the noise of fluorescent lights bothered her. She has problems swallowing and chewing, and has popping or clicking of the jaw. Her ears are itchy, and she has been grinding and clenching her teeth. She had significant eye pain, exhibited sensitivity to light, had challenges with night driving problems, blurry vision, and had dark specks that float in her vision. She did have migraines although not frequently. She had a very stiff neck, a sore spot on the top of her head, pain mid-shoulder when carrying a purse, and pain when writing. She complained of pain with intercourse, muscle cramps and twitches everywhere. She had left foot pain, and very tight hamstrings.

Meagan's TMJ Assessment:

Chief Concern: Meagan's main presenting concern was grinding her teeth, and clicking in her jaw.

- Do you get headaches? Yes
- Do you get migraine headaches? Yes
- Do you frequently have neck aches and stiff neck muscles? Yes
- Do you have chronic shoulder or back pain? Yes
- Do you have trouble sleeping soundly? Yes
- Are your teeth sore when you awaken? Yes
- Have you had your wisdom teeth extracted? Yes
- Do you get headaches in the temporal area? Yes, left

- Do you get headaches in the front or back of your head? Yes
- Do you clench your teeth during the day? Yes
- Do you grind your teeth when asleep? Yes
- When do your pain symptoms get worse? When stressed
- Does anything make it better? Exercise and time off
- Have you been involved in a serious accident? Yes
- Have you ever had a severe blow to the head? Yes
- Any whiplash, neck injury? Yes
- Do you hear clicking or popping in the jaw? Yes
- Do you have difficulty opening wide or yawning? Yes
- Does your jaw ache when opening wide or yawning? Yes
- Are there times when your eyesight blurs? Yes
- Do you get pain in, around or behind either eye? Yes
- Do you have itching or stuffiness in either ear? Yes
- Do you have allergies, sinus problems or snores? No
- Have you been diagnosed with sleep apnea? No

Meagan's Meridian Assessment:

When I asked Meagan which tooth/teeth that thought might be hitting first. She replied that tooth # 27 made contact first when she brings her bottom jaw forward. She says she hits tooth # 18 when she does not bring her bottom jaw forward. Canine tooth # 27, the second incisor on the bottom right frequently tries to keep the bottom jaw forward and when she does this her tooth hits first. Meagan mentioned that she doesn't know why she brings her bottom jaw forward, she did note that It just feels better! Note: By bringing the bottom jaw forward she also pulls the tongue away from the back of her throat and opens her airway and she can breathe better.

Using Meridian Chart: Tooth # 27

Organs: R side of liver, gallbladder, biliary ducts right side
Endocrine: R ovary, R testicle
Vertebrae: Cervical 1,2; Thoracic 8,9,10

Sensory: Anterior R eye
Systems: None
Muscles: R gluteus maximus
Joints: R posterior knee, R hip, R lateral ankle
Sinus: Sphenoid

Using Meridian Chart: Tooth # 18

Organs: L side of large intestine, L lung
Endocrine: None
Vertebrae: Cervical 1,2,5,6,7; Thoracic 2,3,4; Lumbar 4,5
Sensory: Nose
Systems: Arteries
Muscles: L quadriceps
Joints: Radial side of L shoulder, L hand, L elbow, L foot and L big toe
Sinus: Ethmoid

Many of Meagan's symptoms correlated with the symptoms on the meridians.

Meagan's Airway Assessment:

When Meagan's upper palate was measured, it was discovered that only ¾ of the cotton roll would fit across her upper palate. As noted in the case studies of chapter 6, this is indicative of a narrow palate. Meagan reported that she did not sleep well, although she did not report any snoring. She also suffered from restless leg syndromes.

I was not using the airway questionnaire at the time that I assessed Meagan I was just measuring her upper palate of her mouth to determine if there might be a compromised airway.

Treatment:

Meagan is being treated by TMJ dentist Dr Rondeau in London, Ontario. She now has a day and night time dental splint as part of her TMJ treatment.

Case # 3a: Suzzane:

Suzzane is a 72-year-old female who has been experiencing fibromyalgia symptoms for over 20 years. She has 2 tori- which is a bone grown under her tongue. She reports not sleeping well and has difficulty walking.

Suzzane's Fibromyalgia Symptoms:

Suzzane noticed that she seemed to be very attracted by mosquitoes and black flies. She experienced significant fatigue. She had mottled or blotchy skin. She recognized that she was craving carbohydrates. She noticed that she was developing an overgrowth of connective tissue, and prominent nail ridges. She was having overall body aches and pains. She recognized that she was experiencing frequent bouts of frustration. Suzzane felt that she had both an inability to sweat and conversely has extreme night sweats. Suzzane had patches of skin with a painful network of fine veins and capillaries. She had delayed physical pain reaction when very active. She bruises very easily. The fluorescent light bothers Suzanne, and she experiences numbness or tingling. She has had a car accident.

Suzzane's Symptoms Associated with trigger points in the head:

Suzzane had significant motor coordination problems, frequent runny nose and ear pain. She ensured fluctuating blood pressure, as well as dry eyes, nose and mouth. She had popping/clicking of the jaw, and itchy ear. Suzanne had extreme sensitivity to light and had night driving problems. Suzanne had migraines, but was treated successfully with acupuncture. She had a stiff neck, and a sore spot on top of the head.

Symptoms Caused by Fibromyalgia Trigger Points in the Shoulder, Arm, Chest and Back, Buttocks and Groin:

Suzanne experienced pain mid-shoulder when carrying a purse. She has shortness of breath. She often had burning or foul smelling urine, and pain with intercourse. She frequently has low back pain and sciatica.

Symptoms caused by buttocks, leg and foot trigger points:

Suzzane has both upper and lower leg cramps. She has muscle cramps and twitches everywhere. She ensures buckling knees, foot pain, tight hamstrings, restless leg syndrome, a staggering walk and balance problems.

Suzane's TMJ Symptoms

- Do you get headaches? Did have until 18 months ago, relieved with acupuncture
- Do you frequently have neck aches or stiff neck muscles? Yes
- Have you ever had chronic shoulder or back pain? Yes
- Do you have trouble sleeping soundly? Yes
- Have you had wisdom teeth extracted? Yes
- Do you clench or grind your teeth? No
- Where are your pain symptoms worse? Legs, left arm, neck, shoulder back.
- Trauma, whiplash or accident? Yes (car accident hit from front and back 1972) 50 years ago
- Do you have dizziness? Yes
- Does you jaw ever lock? No
- Do you feel or hear clicking the jaw? Yes
- Do you have difficulty opening wide or yawning? Yes
- Does your jaw ache when wide open? Yes
- Have you ever had pain in either jaw joint? Yes
- Do you wear glasses? Yes
- Are there times when your eyesight blurs? Yes
- Do you get pain in, around or behind your eyes? Yes
- Do you have pain in either ear? Yes
- Do you suffer from loss of hearing? No
- Do you have itchiness or stuffiness in either ear? Yes
- Do you have allergies? Yes
- Do you have sinus problems? Yes

- Do you snore at night? Yes
- Have you been diagnosed with sleep apnea? never tested

Medication: Trazadone to sleep, Bisoprol

Suzzane's Meridian Assessment:

When the meridian assessment was done, she notices she was hitting tooth # 7 first which is one of the 4 front teeth.

Organs: R kidneys, R side of bladder, R ovary/testicle, prostate/uterus, rectum/anus
Endocrine: Pineal gland
Vertebrae: Cervical 1,2; Lumbar 2,3; Sacral 3,4,5; Coccyx
Sensory: Nose
Systems: None
Muscles: R subscapularis
Joints: R posterior knee, R sacro-coccygeal, R posterior ankle
Sinus: R frontal & sphenoid

Many of Suzzane's fibromyalgia symptoms and dry eyes and dry mouth relate to this meridian.

Airway:

When Suzanne's upper palate was measured, only 3/4 of the cotton roll fit in her upper palate. It was concluded that her upper palate was narrow. The airway questionnaire was not used when Suzzane was interviewed in February 2021.

Suzzane had 2 large bone growths called tori under her tongue. I questioned if this was affecting if her tongue had enough room in her mouth.

I accompanied Suzzane to the Clearwater Breath Well Sleep Well Clinic. A CAT Scan was done of Suzzane's airway. She was diagnosed with moderate to severe sleep apnea and now has a Vivos dental splint which she wears on her top teeth to expand her upper palate. She turns the screw on the splint every 2 weeks to widen her upper palate, with the goal to increase her airway which was compromised. Suzzane has only had her Vivos splint for 6 months.

You can find out more about results of the Vivos splint at vivos.com or youtube videos on the Vivos splint.

Suzzane had an assessment of the Torri growths under her tongue She will be assessed as her treatment progresses whether these tori will need to be removed.

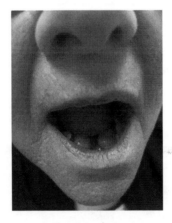

Suzzane's Tori

Case # 4a: Jo-Ellen:

Jo-Ellen Is a 75-year-old woman. Her right jaw was broken by the dentist when he extracted her wisdom teeth in her early 20's. She also had fallen on her back and had received a concussion, and had headaches for years. Jo-Ellen's chief concern has been persistent jaw pain and migraines. She has a major overbite-her bottom teeth are way behind her front teeth. When I suggested that she bring her bottom jaw forward and take a deep breath she was able to take a much deeper breath.

Jo-Ellen's Fibromyalgia Symptoms:

Jo-Ellen often felt debilitating fatigue, and had an intense craving for carbohydrates. She often experienced bouts of frustration, and thick mucus secretions. Jo-Ellen often felt extreme delayed reactions of pain and exhaustion following a too physically active day the previous day. She would often get the shakes when she was hungry, and she bruised easily. She had recent weight loss, she noticed that the noise of fluorescent light bothers her. She has an extreme sensitivity to electromagnetic, electrical storms and full moon/tide pulls. She often experienced numbness or tingling in her jaw.

Symptoms Associate with Trigger Points in the Head:

Jo-Ellen frequently experienced sinus stuffiness, runny nose, trouble swallowing, and ear pain, dry eyes, nose and mouth. She often has problems swallowing and chewing, and has popping or clicking of the jaw. Her ear was often itchy, she usually would grind and clench her teeth. She experienced sensitivity to light, frequent migraines and a painful stiff neck.

Symptoms Caused by Trigger Points in the Shoulder, Arm, Chest and Back, Buttocks and Groin:

Jo-Ellen often had mid-shoulder pain when carrying a purse. She had shortness of breath, frozen shoulder, and chest tightness. Additionally, she had been diagnosed with an irritable bladder and bowel.

Symptoms Caused by Buttocks, Leg, and Foot Trigger Points:

Jo-Ellen has high arches in her feet. She often experiences numbness, hypersensitivity, the feeling of ants crawling under skin on the outer thigh and hip. She also had left foot plantar pain.

Jo-Ellen's TMJ Symptom:

- Do you get migraine headaches? Yes
- Do you frequently have neck aches or stiff neck muscles? Yes
- Have you ever had chronic shoulder or back pain? Yes
- Do you have trouble sleeping soundly? Yes
- Are your jaws tired when you awaken? Yes
- Are your teeth sore when you awaken? No
- Have you had your wisdom teeth extracted? Yes, dentist broke my jaw at this time
- Do you get headaches in the temple area? No
- Do you get headaches in the front of your head? Yes
- Do you clench your teeth during the day? Yes
- Do you grind your teeth when asleep? Yes
- When are your pain symptoms worse? When I overdo it
- Does anything make you feel better? Pain meds
- How often do you take them? Every day
- Have you ever had a severe blow to the head or jaw? Yes
- Are there any foods you avoid eating? Yes
- Do you ever get dizzy? Yes
- Do you ever feel faint? Yes
- Do you never feel nauseated? Yes
- Is there a family history of TMJ problems? No
- Do you have pain in either ear? Yes
- Do you hear ringing or buzzing in your ear? Yes
- Do you have loss of hearing? No
- Do you have allergies? Yes
- Do you have sinus problems? Yes
- Do you snore at night? Yes
- Do you have clicking in your ear? Yes
- Has your jaw ever locked when you were unable to open or close? Yes
- Have you ever had pain in either jaw joint? Yes
- Does your jaw ache when you open wide? Yes
- Do you wear glasses? Yes, for reading

- Are there times when your eyesight blurs? Yes
- Do you get pain in or around or behind your eye? No
- Is your nose stuffy when you don't have a cold? Yes
- Have you ever had a sleep study? No
- Have you been diagnosed with sleep apnea? No

Medication: Thyroxine, B12, Risedronate Curcumin, and multivitamins.

Jo-Ellen's Airway Assessment:

When I assessed Jo-Ellen's palate, I was only able to insert ¾ of a cotton role. I determined that her upper palate is narrow.

Airway questionnaire: Symptoms that Jo- Ellen has:

- Dry lips (usually from mouth breathing)
- TMJ clicking
- Dysphagia (difficulty swallowing due to lack of volume for the tongue within the dental arch)
- High or narrow upper palate
- Chewing cheek
- Dry mouth in the morning
- Drooling during sleep (mouth is open)
- Constantly tired (may be due to anaemia or low oxygen)
- Obstructive sleep apnea
- Severe fatigue after exercise
- Tinnitus (ringing in the ear)
- Fullness in the ear
- Difficulty nasal breathing (has a deviated septum)

Meridian Assessment:

Jo- Ellen thinks she is hitting tooth # 29 first

Tooth # 29 Meridian

Organs: Esophagus, right side of stomach, pancreas, pylorus, pyloric antrum
Endocrine: R mammary glands
Vertebrae: Cervical 1,2; Thoracic 11,12; Lumbar 1
Sensory: Tongue
Systems: Lymph
Muscles: R pectoral major, sternal, hamstrings
Joints: Anterior R hip, anterior R knee, R medial ankle, R jaw
Sinus: R maxillary

Although Jo-Ellen had many of the symptoms on the meridian, she had more symptoms on the left side of her body than her right side.

Jo - Ellen is positive on the TMJ and Airway questionnaire and will be assessed by a TMJ dentist

She is making an appointment with Dr Brock Rondeau. A TMJ and Sleep apnea dentist.

Case # 5a: Sue

Sue is a 75-year-old woman who has had fibromyalgia symptoms since February 2002.

Sue expressed chief concerns of back and leg pain. She has been unable to get a restful sleep, and experiences profound fatigue.

Fibromyalgia Symptoms:

Sue found herself to be very attracted by mosquitoes and black flies. Sue experiences fatigue, exhibits mottled or blotchy skin, and craves carbohydrates. She has body-wide aches and pains. She had realized that she has a very low and frequent frustration tolerance. She often experiences unusual reactions to medications, including antibiotics. She often has thick mucus secretions. She experiences morning sweats, and delayed exhaustion fatigue until the next day if too active physically. She reported often getting a dizzy, faint feeling when hungry. She bruises easily, and has had a recent weight change (gain). She reports that the noise of fluorescent light bothers her. She reports numbness and tingling. She has had numerous surgeries: both knees replaced, right hip replaced, and three back surgeries. She has experienced significant physical trauma: fell down a steep hill in 2018. She broke her arm in three places and had a rotator cuff tear.

Fibromyalgia Symptoms Associated with Trigger Points in the Head:

Sue reports an unusual degree of clumsiness, sinus stuffiness at times, and frequent runny nose. She has fluctuating blood pressure, dry eyes, nose and mouth. She often was grinding and clenching her teeth. She presents as having sensitivity to light, night driving problems, blurry vision, and dark specks that float through her vision. When she reads, she mentions that words jump on the page. Sue also describes a sore spot on top of the head.

Symptoms Caused by Trigger Points in the Shoulder, Arm, Chest and Back, Buttocks and Groin:

Sue often had mid-shoulder pain when carrying a purse, pain when writing, a changing signature, and illegible handwriting. She was often having esophageal reflux, shortness of breath, hypersensitive nipples or breast pain, and chest tightness. There was often intestinal bloating, irritable bladder and bowel. She felt pain with intercourse, had low back pain and sciatica.

Symptoms Caused by Buttocks, Leg and Foot Trigger Points:

She describes that she often stumbles over her own feet. She often has upper and lower leg cramps, foot pain, numbness, hypersensitivity on the outer thigh. She has burning and redness on the inner thigh, a staggering walk and balance problems.

TMJ Questionnaire:

- Do you have headaches or migraines? No
- Do you have frequent neck aches? Yes
- Have you ever had chronic shoulder or back pain? Yes
- Do you have trouble sleeping soundly? Yes
- Are your jaws tired when you awaken? Yes
- Have you had your wisdom teeth extracted? Yes
- Do you clench your teeth during the day? Yes
- Do you clench your teeth at night? Yes
- Do you grind your teeth when asleep? Yes
- When are your symptoms worse? Early a.m. and with exercise
- What makes pain better? Ice sometimes, hot showers, and stretching
- Have you ever had a severe blow to the head? No
- Have you ever had a whiplash? No
- Have you had a serious accident? Yes, a fall
- Do you feel or hear a clicking noise in the jaw joint? Yes
- Has your jaw ever locked? No
- Do you have difficulty opening your mouth wide? Yes
- Have you ever had pain in either jaw joint? Yes
- Do you wear glasses? Yes
- Are there times when your eyesight blurs? Yes
- Do you get pain around or behind the eyes? No
- Do you have pain in your ears? No
- Do you have hearing loss? No
- Do you have itchy ears? Yes
- Do you hear ringing or buzzing in your ears? Yes
- Do you have allergies? Yes, sulpha
- Do you have sinus problems? No
- Is your nose stuffy when you don't have a cold? Yes
- Have you been diagnosed with sleep apnea? Not at time of TMJ assessment
- Have you had a sleep study done at a sleep clinic? No, not at this time

Airway Assessment:

I was not doing an airway questionnaire at this time in assessing fibromyalgia sufferers but I was measuring upper palates. Sue's palate was measured with cotton roll and could only get 3/4 of cotton roll around her upper palate. This would suggest a narrow palate.

Meridian Assessment:

Sue says she is hitting her front teeth first when tapping her teeth together:

Tooth # 9 Left First Incisor, Bladder/Kidney Meridian

Organs: L kidney, bladder, L ovary/testicle, prostate/uterus, rectum/anus
Endocrine: Pineal gland
Vertebrae: Cervical 1,2; Lumbar 2,3; Sacral 3,4,5; Coccyx
Sensory: Nose
Systems: None
Muscles: L neck-flexors, and extensors
Joints: L posterior knee, L sacra-coccygeal, L posterior ankle
Sinus: L frontal and L sphenoid

On returning to Michigan from Florida, Sue made an appointment with Dr Dan Gole, a Head, Neck and Facial Pain Dentist in Hastings, Michigan. He treated her dental issues. She had two high crowns. After one visit, Sue reports starting to sleep better. She now has a TMJ splint as part of her treatment to recovery.

Case Study # 6a: Danielle:

Danielle is a 38-year-old mother of one who had cardiomyopathy after having her now 2-year-old child. She overheard me telling my neighbour, who works in a doctor's office, that I was writing a book on fibromyalgia and she was interested in my findings. She agreed to be interviewed. At the time I did not have the extensive fibromyalgia questionnaire as I do now, but asked about many of the symptoms that I had experienced. I did not measure palates at that time, but I did notice that Danielle was in a crossbite. This condition was familiar to me as I had experienced this while my dental bridge was in place. See illustration below for what a cross bite looks like. The space between the two front teeth should line up to the middle of your bottom teeth, and if they don't you have a crossbite. This is Danielle's crossbite.

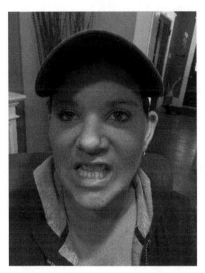

Fibromyalgia Symptoms:

Danielle has shoulder and neck pain, and is unable to turn her head all the way to the left. She has frequent bruising, suffers from a lack of concentration and is often unable to find the right words when speaking. She has fullness and itching in her ears. She reports snoring, being very tired and often falling asleep during the day. She has frequent episodes of sweating at night, blurred vision in her left eye, and panic attacks. She often feels faint, has sciatica, and low back pain. Her fingernails exhibit ridging, and she often has cold hands and feet. Her tongue scalloped around the edges. Her heels often feel as though they are burning and she frequently has difficulty getting comfortable. She often experiences constipation, and indigestion. Her mouth often feels bruised after brushing her teeth. She has had many sore throats. Her balance was off, she often ran into walls. The left ankle twists easily, She reports that she would sometimes catch her big toe when she walks. Her right foot is flat footed.

TMJ Health Questionnaire:

- Do you have headaches? Yes
- Do you have migraine headaches? Yes
- Do you frequently have neck aches or stiff neck muscles? Yes
- Have you ever had chronic shoulder or back pain? Yes
- Do you have trouble sleeping soundly? Yes
- Are you jaw tired when you awaken? Yes
- Are your teeth sore when you awaken? Yes
- Are your wisdom teeth extracted? Yes
- Do you get headaches in the right or left temple areas? Yes
- Do you get headaches in the front and back of your head? Yes
- Do you clench your teeth during the day? Yes
- Do you clench your teeth during the night? Yes
- Do you grind your teeth when asleep? Yes
- When are your symptoms worse? At night
- Does anything make you feel better? Relax and lay down
- How often do you take medication for relief of pain? Day
- Have you ever been in a serious accident? No
- Have you ever had a whiplash? No
- Have you ever had a severe blow to the head? Yes
- Does your jaw feel tired after a big meal? Yes
- Do you ever get dizzy? Yes
- Do you ever feel faint? Yes
- Do you ever feel nauseated? Yes
- Is there a family history of TMJ? No
- Do you feel or hear the clicking of jaw joint? Yes
- Has your jaw ever locked open or closed? No
- Does your jaw ache when you open wide? Yes
- Do you wear contacts or glasses? Yes

- Are there times when your eyesight blurs? Yes
- Do you get pain in or around or behind either eye? Yes
- Do you have pain in your ears? No
- Do you suffer from loss of hearing? Yes
- Do you hear ringing in either ear? Yes
- Do you have allergies? No
- Do you have sinus problems? No
- Do you snore at night? Yes
- Is your nose stuffy when you don't have a cold? Yes
- Have you ever had a sleep study, or diagnosed with sleep apnea? No

Medications: fluid pill, arthritic medication, stomach medication, muscle relaxant, pain pills and psoriasis medication, and anti- inflammatory

Meridian Chart:

Tooth # 13 Second Premolar, Meridian Large Intestine

Organs: L lung, large intestine on the left, L bronchi
Endocrine: thymus
Vertebrae: Cervical 1,2,5,6,7; Thoracic 2,3,4; Lumbar 4,5
Sensory: Left side of nose
Systems: L breast
Muscles: L diaphragm, L pectoralis major clavicular
Joints: Radial side of left shoulder, L hand, L elbow, L foot and L big toe
Sinus: Ethmoid

Danielle is moving and plans to go see a dentist about her crossbite. She had beautiful teeth with few fillings, but her dental alignment needed to be assessed.

Case Study # 7a: Kim:

Kim is a 55-year-old woman who exhibits a severe overbite. Her bottom teeth are barely visible behind her top teeth. She presents with many stomach issues, and the left side of her jaw clicks. When Kim was assessed using the cotton roll test for assessing her palate, it was determined that her palate is very narrow. As mentioned, she exhibits a severe overbite, and reports that her tongue does not seem to fit in her mouth. When I suggested that she move her bottom jaw forward, she said she could breathe more deeply. She mentioned that she wished that her bottom jaw was forward all the time.

Fibromyalgia Questionnaire - Symptoms:

Kim experiences extreme fatigue, exhibits mottled or blotchy skin, and frequently craves carbohydrates. She often has extreme sweating at night, and has patches of skin with a painful network of fine veins and capillaries. She seems to be extremely susceptible to infection. Like many other individuals with fibromyalgia, she experiences delayed fatigue reaction when active physically. She often has extreme sensitivity to the noise of fluorescent lights. She has electromagnetic sensitivity-affected by electrical storms. She often has numbness or tingling. She reports having several serious illnesses and trauma: car accident, endometriosis, and physical injuries.

Symptoms Associated with the Head:

Kim seems to have an unusual degree of clumsiness. She reports sinus stuffiness, frequent runny nose, and trouble swallowing. She has ear pain, dry eyes, nose and mouth. She mentioned that she sometimes had problems swallowing and chewing. She had red or tearing eyes, popping or clicking of the jaw, and itchy ears. She noticed that she does grind and clench her teeth, and has unexplained toothache. She has left eye pain, and that night driving had become a problem. She had double and blurry vision, and dark specks that float in her vision. She experiences frequent headaches, stiff neck and dizziness when she turns her head. She has a sore spot on top of the head and has difficulty turning head to the left.

Symptoms Trigger Points in Shoulder, Arm, Chest and Back:

Kim has mid-shoulder pain when carrying a purse. She sometimes has esophageal reflux. Kim sometimes experiences shortness of breath, and exhibits hypersensitivity on the left side of her body. She has great pain, and chest tightness on the left side. She often has Irritable bladder and bowel symptoms, and sometimes has strong smelling urine. She has experienced menstrual problems-endometriosis and low back pain.

Symptoms Caused by Buttocks, Leg, and Foot Trigger Point:

Kim has weak ankles, and often stumbles over her own feet. She has both upper and lower leg cramps. She has foot pain, tight hamstrings, a staggering walk and balance problems. Her toe often catches when walking.

TMJ Health Questionnaire:

- Do you get headaches? Yes
- Do you get migraine headaches? No
- Do you frequently have neck aches or stiff neck muscles? Yes
- Have you ever had chronic shoulder or back pain? Yes
- Do you have trouble sleeping soundly? Yes
- Are your jaws tired when you awaken? Yes
- Are your teeth sore when you awaken? Yes
- Have your wisdom teeth been extracted? Yes
- Do you get headaches in the R and L temporal areas? Yes
- Do you get headaches in the front or back of the head? Yes
- Do you clench your teeth during the day? Yes
- Do you clench your teeth at night? Yes
- When are your pain symptoms worse? Constant during the day

- Does anything make you feel better? Not really
- Do you take medication for pain? Yes, Tylenol
- Have you ever had a severe blow to the head or jaw? Yes
- Any whiplash injuries? Yes
- Have you ever been involved in any serious accidents? Yes, I was T-boned on right side 25 yrs ago, no broken bones, soft tissue damage and whiplash
- Does your jaw feel tired after a big meal? Yes
- Are there any foods you avoid eating? Yes
- Do you ever get dizzy? Yes
- Do you ever feel faint? Yes
- Do you ever feel nauseated? Yes
- Is there a family history of TMJ? No
- Do you feel or hear clicking or popping in either jaw? Yes, sometimes
- Has your jaw ever locked when you are able to open or close? Yes, sometimes
- Do you have difficulty opening wide? Yes
- Have you ever had pain in either jaw joint? Yes
- Does your jaw ache when you open wide? Yes
- Do you wear glasses or contacts? Yes
- Are there times when your eyesight blurs? Yes
- Do you get pain in, around or behind either eye? Yes, left eye
- Do you have pain in your ear? Yes
- Do you suffer from any loss of hearing? Yes
- Do you have itchiness or stuffiness in either ear? Yes
- Do you hear ringing, buzzing, in either ear? Yes
- Do you have allergies? Yes
- Do you have sinus problems? Yes
- Do you snore at night? Yes
- Is your nose stuffy when you don't have a cold? Yes
- Have you had a sleep study or been diagnosed with sleep apnea? No

Kim feels that she hits tooth # 13 first and many of her symptoms are on this meridian.

Tooth # 13 Second Premolar, Meridian Large Intestine

Organs: L lung, large intestine on the left, L bronchi
Endocrine: thymus
Vertebrae: Cervical 1,2,5,6,7; Thoracic 2,3,4; Lumbar 4,5
Sensory: Left side of nose
Systems: L breast
Muscles: L diaphragm, L pectoralis major clavicular
Joints: Radial side of left shoulder, L hand, L elbow, L foot and L big toe
Sinus: Ethmoid

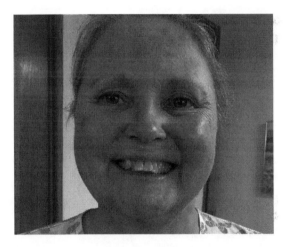

Kim had a high narrow upper palate. I could only get about less than 3/4 of the cotton roll in when I measured her upper palate.

Note: Any individual that can only see 4 to 6 teeth when the person smiles probably has a narrow upper palate. I refer to this as a narrow smile.

The narrow upper palate is not only in adults but also in children, as we saw with Mya in chapter 6.

Kim plans to get treatment when finances are available.

Chapter 8

Dental Cases That May Surprise You

Different outcome requires different thinking.
~ Thomas M Rau, MD,
Medical Director, Paracelsus Clinic, Switzerland

The following dental cases are derived from the practices of dentists that I have had an opportunity to meet during my dental journey and research to help others. They include Dr Ralph Garcia: TMJ Dentist, Tampa, Florida; Dr Dan Gole: Head, Neck and Facial Pain Dentist Hastings Michigan, Dr Brock Rondeau: Orthodontist TMJ, and Snoring Dentist, London, Ontario; and Dr Felix Liao: a Holistic Mouth and Airway Dentist from Falls Church, Virginia. All of these dentists have lectured on dental and airway issues all over the world. I find it amazing that a nurse from Sombra, Ontario, Canada has been able to find and get to know these dentists with such a wide range of knowledge about the jaw, airway, and teeth. After talking with them, they have allowed me to share some of their dental cases. I share these cases to highlight that not all dentists have a drill/ fill philosophy and practice. These cases are not reflective of what has been, nor what is taught in dental school. It is important to recognize that one cannot expect a general dentist will have knowledge of these amazing cases, nor how to treat them in these ways.

Dr Dan Gole D.D.S.: Hastings, Michigan. Head Neck and Facial Pain Dentist, Myofascial Certification, American Orthodontics, American Academy of Pain Management, American Academy of Orofacial Pain

As mentioned in chapter 1 and 2, Dr Gole is the dentist that saved my life. After seeing five dentists in Canada, he was the one who recognized that my dental bridge had not been placed correctly. When he removed my dental bridge, the teeth that the dentist filed to attach my bridge were not straight. This caused my bridge to sit too close to my cheek. When he removed my dental bridge, all of my fibromyalgia symptoms went away except my migraine headaches. I received treatment for my migraines later by Dr Rondeau. Dr Gole is the dentist that I refer to any of the Michigan patients with fibromyalgia that I interview.

Dr Gole's Fibromyalgia Case Studies from one of his newsletters:

Case # 1

Kelly is a 38-year-old female who has a wide array of chief complaints: 1) Pain all over, 2) fatigue, 3) dizziness, 4) tendonitis, 5) stomach problems, 6) Vision problems, 7) pleurisy, and 8) migraine headaches all of which started in the last 7 months.

Kelly had been given multiple diagnoses from different practitioners: Lupus Erythematosus (LE), Temporomandibular Joint Dysfunction (TMD), migraine headaches, and tendonitis to name a few. The Mayo clinic had diagnosed her as having Fibromyalgia Syndrome (FMS): According to the World Health Organisation the official diagnosis of fibromyalgia is defined as a painful, but not articular (not present in joints) condition predominantly involving muscles, and as the most common cause of chronic widespread musculoskeletal pain.

Kelly presented to us (Dr Gole's practice), with a bite splint that was out of balance. She had been diagnosed by a previous dentist with TMJ. Stress levels were high in her life. Her fingers were going numb, her eyes were bloodshot and the eyelids were twitching. All medical testing was negative. Balancing the splint helped with her headaches and neck pain but not with the fatigue. Kelly was searching for answers. She went to another dental office and had all of her amalgam (silver-mercury) fillings removed. Huge composite (tooth coloured fillings) were placed in all of the remaining back teeth. The dentist had also extracted all the teeth with root canals and performed surgery to remove possible bone cavitation (NICO lesions). After all of the dental interventions were complete, her symptoms remained unchanged.

Kelly had her bite balanced, and one last abscessed tooth removed. At that point, her mouth was restored. Utilising the RFV Technique (Resultant Force Vector Technique / muscle testing) to identify the body dysfunction, Kelly is now pain free, functioning well, and has all of her symptoms under control.

Case # 2

Patient is a 35-year-old female patient suffering for five years with the following symptoms: achy, stiff, painful muscles throughout the body, headache, fatigue, disturbed sleep, inability to concentrate, depression, food allergies, bruises easily, irritable bowel syndrome, hands are constantly white and cold, irritable, and weak muscles making exercising excruciating.

The cause of these symptoms is unclear after her last pregnancy, however she was eventually diagnosed with fibromyalgia. The stiffness and pain deep within the muscles makes even simple tasks seem difficult. Emotional tension and hormonal swings aggravate the knotting in the muscle. "Pills and learn to live with it "were the suggested conservative options along with exercise and Physical Therapy.

Treatment: RFV Analysis revealed tender muscles throughout the body. Functional testing showed a positive link to the teeth, indicating that favourable changes could be made through a dental perspective.

135

Phase 1: Treatment consisted of an oral orthotic appliance (splint), and physical modalities eliminated 85 to 90% of the patients' symptoms in eight weeks.

Phase 2: Treatment using the RF Technique, put the patient back on her own teeth in four weeks. "Fine tuning the bite has made life enjoyable again. A six month post-treatment evaluation shows a 95 to 98% reduction in symptoms.

Dr Gole's: ADHD Case Study from one of his newsletters:

Case #3

This patient is a nine-year-old boy that teachers felt was out of control. He was diagnosed with attention deficit disorder (ADD), and Ritalin was prescribed to control his behaviour. While on medication, this child lost his creativity and had begun to hate school. A number of strategies and approaches were used to try and help this young man: counselling, switching schools and trying a different physician, who changed the diagnosis to ADHD (attention deficit/hyperactivity disorder) were all equally, minimally effective. His frustrated parents researched the internet and found that Ritalin is prescribed in Michigan more than any other state in the nation. The parents found this very concerning, given that it was minimally effective.

Examination revealed greater muscle tension when this patient sat down than when he was standing. The referring chiropractor found a strong dental connection. His bite was off, and the provocation testing was positive.

Treatment involved functional appliance therapy and bite balancing. The dental stress was diminished. After two months, this child turned into a model student: His grades went from Cs and Ds to As and Bs. Classroom participation and attention improved. The mother is feeling blessed that her son is doing well and that he is drug free.

Dr Felix Liao D.D.S.: Falls Church, Virginia: Holistic Mouth Dentist: Certified Biological Dentist, Mastership in the Academy of Dentistry, Board Certified by the American Board of General Dentistry

From his book: ***Six-Foot Tiger, Three Foot Cage,*** Holistic Mouth Solution for Sleep Apnea, Deficient Jaws, and Related Complication

Case #1: Tourette's Syndrome:

Turning an "impaired mouth" into a" holistic mouth" can be an effective solution to resolve many symptoms in and around the mouth and often throughout the body. In Case 1, we will consider Luke. He was a nine-year-old boy, who had an overbite, and exhibited facial tics from Tourette syndrome. He had buck teeth, chronic mouth breathing, and low energy. All of these oral complications interfered with his health and schooling. A year after starting treatment, Luke was 100 percent free of any facial tics. Two and a half years later, he became a straight-A student, taking advanced math and language arts courses and playing tennis.

"I drove four hours each way (every other month) over these three years," says Luke's dad. "I'm really proud that he's doing so well."

Luke says " I feel I have lots of energy, and it's easier to learn now and I feel happier."

When the tongue's habitat is too small, it is forced into the throat, backing the airway and causing stress from oxygen deficiency day and night.

What if Luke were to graduate, go to work, and start a family without ever having his impaired mouth treated? Imagine the harmful effects it would have on his quality of life - not to mention his health-care cost!

Dr Liao. Holistic Mouth Dentist:

Case #2:

Smithy, is a 36-year-old woman who presented with a toothache. During the triage, she related to Dr. Liao other symptoms that had been bothering her every day for years: pain in her mouth and gums, random gurgling sounds in her stomach, constant tiredness, and neck, shoulder and wrist pain.

The doctor suspected an impaired mouth and airway obstruction. Upon examination and testing, her "Epworth Sleepiness Score" (an accepted self-survey for sleep apnea) was 14—well about the threshold of 10—which suggested sleep apnea. Her CAT scan showed her airway was in the red zone - the danger zone — and thus susceptible to collapse during sleep.

After a detailed consultation, Smithy elected to start treatment using oral appliances to redevelop her jaws, bite and airway to help her sleep better. She was instructed to wear her appliance fourteen to sixteen hours a day, included when she slept but excluding office hours. Four months later, Smithy reported a 50 % drop in her neck, shoulder and carpal-tunnel pain, a 60% drop in her stress-related mouth pain, a 70 % drop in her stomach symptoms and an 80 % drop in fatigue.

Seven months after starting a personalized oral-appliance therapy, Smithy reported that her Epworth Sleepiness Score had dropped from 14 to 9 and she was sleeping better and dreaming more (a sign of deep sleep).

Smithy's case shows that the mouth structure plays a role in symptoms inside, around, and beyond the mouth. It should be noted that Smithy had immaculate oral hygiene. She was just stuck with <u>a structurally impaired mouth.</u>

An "impaired mouth" negatively impacts health while a "holistic mouth" promotes total health. Redeveloping an impaired mouth into a Holistic Mouth can improve many symptoms naturally and unexpectedly. This is a consistent outcome in my (Dr. Liao) experience.

Dr Ralph Garcia,D.D.S. TMJ Dentist Tampa, Florida Academy of Dentistry International, Fellow International College of Craniomandibular Orthopaedics, Fellow American Academy of Pain Management, Board Certified International Assoc. for Orthodontics.

Summary of 3 cases:

Case #1: Dr. Ralph Garcia

The patient is a 27-year-old female that came to my practice in Tampa but is a student who attends Syracuse University. She presented in my office suffering from severe migraine headaches. She had been prescribed Sumatriptan for a number of years and she could not tolerate all of the side effects any longer. She also had other symptoms: Jaw pain, neck pain, facial pain, clicking/popping in the joints, and ear stuffiness.

We delivered an orthopaedic repositioning appliance (ORA) and night/muscle relaxation appliance on Aug 16, 2020 and adjusted the appliances once before she went back to Syracuse University.

We did not see her again until Nov 3, 2020. She had been symptom free for four (4) months when she returned to our office.

We started Phase II treatment immediately upon her return and completed her Phase II treatment, which included orthopaedic and orthodontics (). We completed her Phase II June 2022 and she has remained symptoms free throughout her treatment.

Definition:

Orthopaedics refer to the branch of dentistry concerned with conditions involving realignment and development of the jaw and musculo/skeletal system

Orthodontics: the treatment of irregularities in the teeth and jaw

Case # 2: Dr. Ralph Garcia

The patient is a 58-year-old white male who was referred to our office for severe pain which his Michigan Dentist attributed to an abscess tooth. He indicated that he was here to have it taken care of at my office, since he had transferred to Tampa from Michigan.

We tested his teeth with percussion, a vitalometer, sensitivity to heat and cold, and we did a full mouth x-ray. All these tests were negative for abscess.

Examination and history indicated that all the signs and symptoms suggested a more accurate diagnosis of severe temporomandibular disorder (TMD). He presented with severe maxillary and mandibular buttressing, severe deep bite, ear stuffiness, hearing loss, facial pain, and clicking jaw joints. We constructed and delivered an orthopaedic repositioning appliance (ORA) and night appliance/muscle relaxation appliance.

After using the appliances for two weeks he was at maximum medical improvement (MMI): in other words, the patient was completely symptom free. His hearing returned to normal and his jaw pain, facial pain, and TMJ clicking had been resolved. The patient had prior extensive dental procedures, with many crowns and fixed bridges. We had to perform a full mouth rehabilitation, and created a corrected (therapeutic) jaw position. The post treatment has allowed the patient to remain symptom free for over eight years.

Case # 3: Dr. Ralph Garcia

A four-year-old male child presented with a diagnosis of Tourette's syndrome from both his paediatrician and neurologist. The mother was very upset when she told them both that the tic got worse when he was eating and both doctors said that the two were unrelated.

When the mother relayed the story to me, I got excited and told her that I felt we could help her child. Upon examination, the child had an anterior and posterior cross bite, which indicated to me that the trigeminal system was under stress.

We constructed a Quad-Helix dental appliance with occlusal pads to centre the mandible on the cranium. His tics disappeared the moment we gave him the appliance. He has remained tic free for 24 years.

Please find the link to the video on YouTube "Meet Jonathan, A Tourette's Success Story"
https://www.youtube.com/watch?v=OdQDJqoHFBU&t=6s

Dr Brock Rondeau, D.D.S. I.B.O., D.A.B.C.P., D-A.C.S.D.D., D.A.B.D.S.M., A.B.C.D.S.M. Medicine TMJ Dentist, Orthodontist, and Sleep and Airway Dentist, London Ontario

Dr Rondeau is the dentist that treated my migraine headaches by bringing my bottom jaw forward with a splint (this pulled my tongue forward and opened up my airway, as well as pulled the condyle away from the nerves and blood vessels in my jaw). He did my orthodontics, (braces on my teeth) which resulted in me being free of migraines and allowed me to sleep better. He is the dentist that I refer all of the fibromyalgia, ADHD, and migraine sufferers to that I interview. He is a brilliant dentist, who lectures to other dentists, but can also explain the treatment to patients so that they can easily understand.

Case # 1: Dr. Brock Rondeau

The patient was a fifty-two (52)-year-old male who presented with the following TMJ symptoms as recorded on the TMJ Health Questionnaire:

- Headaches, front of head
- Clenching
- Bruxism (teeth grinding at night)
- Clicking jaw
- Problems sleeping
- History of severe blow to head
- Snores
- Had a sleep study, diagnosed with severe sleep apnea

He further presented a medical history as follows: Patient has diabetes, had shortness of breath, and frequent snoring. Additionally, he was under psychiatric treatment for Bipolar disorder.

Additional medical testing included a HOSPITAL SLEEP STUDY, PSG (POLYSOMNOGRAM). He had an AHI (Apnea Hypopnea Index) of 30 times per hour: which means that this patient stops breathing 30 times per hour all night, and that his Oxygen desaturation was consistently below 90% for 55 minutes. For a healthy person, Oxygen in the blood should average 96%. Oxygen desaturation is a very serious health problem.

EPWORTH SLEEPINESS SCALE as seen in chapter 4: This patient had a score of 12 when this test was administered. This score indicates extreme daytime fatigue and requires medical attention. Patients who score at this level, should be referred to a hospital, private sleep clinic or home sleep study for assessment. Sleep studies must be reviewed, and a diagnosis determined by a sleep specialist.

INITIAL HOSPITAL SLEEP STUDY: Patient experienced extreme daytime fatigue, has diabetes. He and his partner had to have separate bedrooms. He was diagnosed with severe obstructive sleep apnea. At the time, the treatment prescribed was a CPAP. The patient reported being unable to wear CPAP. Unfortunately there was no follow up appointment. Patient could not wear CPAP and had severe sleep apnea. He reported feeling that the medical profession had abandoned him as his health deteriorated.

American Academy of Sleep Recommend - Oral appliances are recommended if patients cannot tolerate CPAP.

This patient was not able to tolerate the CPAP. Dr. Rondeau made him an oral appliance called Somnodent Appliance which moves his lower jaw forward, opens the airway so he can breathe at night. This oral appliance solved his snoring, sleep apnea as well as TM Dysfunction by bringing the lower jaw forward. **Patient then went to the hospital for another sleep study.** His wife also reported that because he was much quieter in the bedroom she now sleeps in the same room after many years apart.

Pretreatment: He looks exhausted and very unhappy. **Post treatment he** looks much younger, more energetic and much happier.

Everyone deserves to get a good night's sleep. As a doctor of dentistry, I was fortunate to be able to significantly improve not only his sleep but his overall health.

This patient highlights the importance of dentists who treat these patients being knowledgeable in both TM Dysfunction and Sleep Disorders. Many TMD patients have sleep problems, and many patients who suffer from snoring and who have sleep apnea also may have TMD problems. These issues are rarely mutually exclusive.

I have enclosed a copy of the following:

TMJ Health Questionnaire (copy in chapter 3)
Patients should fill out this form. If they answer yes to a number of symptoms they need to seek treatment with a dentist with special training in treating

TMD. I personally am a Diplomate in the American Academy of Craniofacial Pain.

Epworth Sleepiness Scale (copy in chapter 4)

This scale is an excellent indication of just how tired the patient is during the daytime. Normal score is 4-5. If the score is over 10 the patient needs medical attention usually because they have sleep apnea. Any score over 10 the patient needs to go to a dentist with special training in treating sleep disorders. I personally have a Diplomate in the American Academy of Dental Sleep Medicine.

Any score over 10 means the patient has significant daytime sleepiness and needs to get either a hospital sleep study, private sleep clinic sleep study or home sleep study in a dental office.

All sleep studies must be diagnosed by a sleep specialist.

Case # 2: TMD CASE Dr Brock Rondeau:

Patient is a 20-year-old female who presented with temporomandibular dysfunction. She had completed orthodontic treatment four years previously, and was in severe pain. Her orthodontic treatment was performed due to irregularities in her teeth and jaw.

The TMJ Health Questionnaire indicated that she was experiencing the following symptoms:

- Headaches
- Neck aches
- Clenching (teeth grinding)
- Bruxing
- Clicking jaw
- Jaw Locking

She had been to her regular dentist and he made her the standard upper flat plane night guard which had made her symptoms worse.

A standard night guard should not be used in a patient whose jaw is dislocated. We know that this is the case, by her TMJ (jaw joint) clicking when she opens and closes her mouth.

Diagnosis: Stage 2 Internal Derangement noise in jaw joint: Clicking, Intermittent locking, Pain:

Patients who wear the standard upper or lower night guard sometimes go to Stage 3: Lock Jaw, where their jaw has limited opening and can only open with one finger between the teeth and are in intense pain. This patient had not progressed to this stage. It was imperative to prevent this from happening.

Dr Brock Rondeau wrote an article on the problems with patients wearing the standard night guard entitled, ***"Why the Fabrication of Occlusal Night Guards May be Detrimental to the Overall Health of the Patient."***

Readers who would like a copy of Dr Brock Rondeau's article can email: contactus@ortho-tmj.com.

Another major problem with a flat night guard is that it encourages the patient to clench and grind their teeth more. This contributes to muscle pain and headaches. **Dentists are advised not to prescribe flat night guards for patients who have clicking jaws.**

Tomogram X-Rays of the TMJ revealed that the patient's condyles (top of the lower jawbone) were too far back when the patient closed on their back teeth. When the condyles are too far posterior they compress the nerves between the condyle and the ear. This causes numerous ear symptoms, including:
- Ringing in the ears
- Ear pain
- Stuffiness in ears

This constellation of symptoms supports the diagnosis of TMJ Dysfunction. Another excellent way to help make the diagnosis is to utilize a device called the Joint Vibration Analysis. This device analyses the noises or vibrations within the TMJ: No joint in the body is supposed to make noise on movement. Normal noise or vibrations with the Joint Vibration Analysis device is 20 or less. When measured with this device, the patient has an extremely noisy TMJ.

TREATMENT PLAN: PHASE 1

1. Lower Repositioning Splint, Daytime:

A splint was designed so the patient cannot click when they open and close their jaw. The literature reports that if one can eliminate the click, then there can be a reduction of jaw symptoms by 94%. Standard night guards do not eliminate clicking of the jaw.

The lower repositioning splint is not flat like the standard night guard. It is an indexed splint that repositions the lower jaw forward in a position such that the jaw does not click when the patient opens and closes their mouth.

A Tomogram X-Ray was taken of the TMJ when the patient was wearing the lower daytime splint. The X-ray confirms that there was now more space between the back of the condyle (top of the lower jaw bone) and the ear. The condyle was no longer compressing on the nerves and blood vessels between the condyle and the ear when the patient bit on her back teeth, and when she swallowed 2,000 times per day. This confirmed that the splint had put the lower jaw in the ideal position.

2. Upper Night Guard to prevent clenching and grinding:

In this phase of the treatment, a splint was made that repositioned the condyle down and forward. At night it is important that the patient wears an appliance that prevents them from clenching and grinding. The design of this patient's night guard is different from the daytime splint. When the patient tries to get their teeth together the back teeth should not touch. The patient cannot clench or grind their teeth at night. This prevents the patient waking up in the morning with headaches. The design of the upper night guard only allowed the front teeth to touch. The Tomogram X-ray revealed that the lower jaw was too far back when the patient bit on her back teeth. To help prevent the patient's jaw from falling back at night, The design of the night guard has a ramp at the front that keeps the lower jaw forward. To help prevent soreness to the lower front teeth. In addition, there was a clear plastic retainer (like Invisalign) to distribute the biting forces more evenly over all the lower teeth. The combination of both the lower splint and the upper night guard completely eliminated the symptoms of TM Dysfunction.

At the end of Phase I, stabilization of the TMJ one of two things can happen:

The bite does not change: the clicking is eliminated, and there are no further TMJ symptoms: These patients are very fortunate and no longer have to continue to wear the lower splint during the daytime. It will be necessary to keep wearing the upper night guard nightly, to keep the lower jaw from falling back and to keep the disc in the correct position. This will prevent the clicking jaw from coming back with all its associated unpleasant symptoms.

If the bite changes: This does happen from time to time. The patient may need additional orthodontic treatment, and may need braces or clear aligners to restore the bite to normal so the patient can chew. When the bite changes there is a space between the back teeth so the patient must wear the lower splint or the patient cannot eat.

To correct the patient's bite, as with this patient, it was necessary to move on to:

Phase II, Orthodontic treatment. Although she had previously had orthodontic treatment, there was a need to redo the work because of the alteration in the bite. When completed the patient no longer had any temporomandibular dysfunction (TMD) symptoms.

End Result: A happy pain free patient

I believe these cases show that there are knowledgeable dentists that can help not only fibromyalgia but other medical conditions. You need to research the dentists in your area and find one that can help you. It is not a quick fix, but it is possible to get better. All of the people that I have interviewed with fibromyalgia also had TMJ dysfunction. Finding a good TMJ dentist who has the proper equipment such as joint vibrational analysis and tomography would be a good place to start. A holistic mouth dentist if you can find one is another option, I would try first. These professionals can address the airway and TMJ issues often associated with fibromyalgia.

I hope that I have provided you with the knowledge for you to get started on a recovery to better health.

Glossary

Amitriptyline: An antidepressant with sedative properties. Affects certain chemical messengers that communicate between brain cells and helps to regulate mood. It is often used to treat depression. In small doses it is often used to treat sleep disturbances and fibromyalgia.

Brux/Bruxation: the motion of subconsciously grinding or clenching teeth and jaws.

Cafergot: Medication (ergotamine and caffeine) used to treat migraine. This medication can be either in pill or suppository form.

Condyle of the jaw: A cartilage growth site in the mandible(jaw) that allows elongation of the jaws arms. The rounded upper end of the lower jaw, which allows movement in the lower part of the jaw joint.

Crepitation: the grating sound of two ends of a broken bone rubbing together

Decadron (Dexamethasone) is a strong steroid and anti-inflammatory used to relieve inflammation in parts of the body. Used to decrease swelling associated with tumours of the spine and brain. Also used to treat eye inflammation. Can be administered in pill form, tablet form, infusion or topically by lotion.

Imitrex (Sumaytripan): used to treat symptoms of migraine headaches, (severe, throbbing headaches that sometimes are accompanied by nausea and sensitivity to sound and light. Can be administered by infusion or injection.

Malocclusion: which means an imperfect positioning of the teeth in the jaw.

Meridian Lines: In the context of medical/holistic terms, and based in Chinese medicine, they are the energy network of the body. The lines are the channels by which our energy flows, transporting the energy throughout the body.

Sjogren's Syndrome: This disorder occurs when the body's white blood cells mistakenly attack moisture-production glands. It causes inflammation and a significant decrease in the quality and quantity of the types of moisture that are produced.

Temporomandibular Joint Disorder (TMJ or TMD): Pain and dysfunction in the side hinge and muscles connecting the jaw to the skull. It can be unilateral or bilateral.

Narcolepsy: A neurological disorder that affects the brain's ability to control sleepfulness and wakefulness. Characterized by unintentionally falling asleep while engaging in normal activities throughout the day.

Appendix

Education for Meridians:

Google Reinhold-Voll
Dr. Voll also researched the TCM idea that teeth are energetically connected to organs. Numerous dental charts depicting the interrelationship between teeth and organs have now been published.

drdawn.net Holistic Health Alternatives
She did her doctoral thesis on the dental organ connection and wrote the Book Let the Tooth be Known. She also developed a meridian dental chart

meridiantoothchart.com see how each tooth relates to an organ
rejuvdentist.com
dentistry4health.org
juliandental.com
https://www.noelckdds.com/meridian-tooth-chart/
naturaldentistassociation.com
brunodentistry.com

YouTube
Meridians - The Tooth/Body Connection. Dawn Ewing, RDH. PHD.

TMJ Information:

YouTube
Treatment Options for TMJ Pain /Joint Disorder - Vivos DNA and Homeoblock Appliances

Many Vivos YouTube videos - just search

Rondeau Seminars
Introduction to Diagnosis and Treatment of TM Dysfunction

TMJ Explanation & Therapy Dr Brian Mills

My TMJ Experience TMJ Treatments, Symptoms,Neck Pain, Scams and Surgery
TMD Tip and what helped Dominic Phillip

Web: www.TMJ.org

Education for Sleep and Airway:

YouTube
Dr Ben Miraglia Connecting Sleep Disordered Breathing and ADD/ADHD
(This is true for adults too)

Sleep Apnea and Breathing Vivos Invisible No More Show

Dr Felix Liao - Welcome to Holistic Mouth Solutions
(This dentist is an amazing airway dentist) a must watch

Connecting the Dots Between Your Mouth Structure and Total Health /Dr Felix Liao

The Neurological Consequence of a Misfit Mouth on Sleep Jerald Simmons
Airway Chat #26 with Dr Ben Miraglia: Overview of Airway Dentistry

Dentists That Can Help Fibromyalgia Patients by Treating TMJ or Airway

Dr Brock Rondeau DDS London Ontario. 519-455-4110

Dr Sylvia Bakabanian DDS Ottawa Ontrario. 613-230-2626

Dr Robert Rousseau DDS Bloomfield Hills Michigan. 248-642-5471

Dr Javana Rae Cosner DDS Battle Creek Michigan. 269-962-5774

Dr Dan Gole DDS Hasting Michigan. 269-953-3050

Dr White DDS Bright White Dental, Manton Michigan. 231-272-0899

Dr Ralph Garcia DDS Tampa Florida. 813-245-9452

Dr Felix Liao DDS Falls Church Virginia. 703-385-6425

Dr Paul DDS Breathwell Sleepwell Clinic, Clearwater Florida. 727-458-5778

Dr Xiauyan Dai DDS Ashton Pennsylvania. 448-716-8806

Dr Doris A Ferres DDS Vero Beach Florida. 772-567-1011

Dr Anthony Huang DDS Vancouver BC. 604-876-9228

Dr Eric Armakan Virginia. 240-660-0954 Frenectomy Specialist (tongue tie release)

Dr Sherry Salartash Falls Church Virgina. 703-447-5829
.

Dr Nemie Sirlian DDS South Plainfield New Jersey. 908-753-5000

Dr Gene Sambataro DDS Julian Center for Comprehensive Dentistry, Ellicott City Maryland. 410-964-3118

Dr Jeff Yelle DDS Mountain Wellness Dentistry Monument Co. 719-488-2375

Natural Dentist Assoc. North Bethesda. MD. 301-273-1815

Centra Dental, Houston Texas. 832-289-8803

Go to vivos.com and look up Vivos provider locator
(there are many dentists on the list)

Otherwise look for an airway, mouth dentist. AMD dentist
TMJ Dentist who do repositioning splints NOT flat plane splints

About the Author

Linda Harris, R.N., BScN., W.O.C.N., certified TMJ Assistant is a Canadian nurse who loves to uncover the reasons behind a person's physical symptoms.

After having fibromyalgia and migraine headaches herself she found the secret to the root cause of her problem: her TMJ, compromised airway and a bite that was off. Once these problems were addressed, her symptoms disappeared and she regained her health.

Once she felt better, Linda started interviewing people with fibromyalgia, and TMJ.

During her research she attended many dental conferences and became a certified TMJ Assistant. This increased her knowledge of the TMJ (temporomandibular joint) fibromyalgia, compromised airways, and migraine headaches.

Her dental journey allowed her to meet some of the most amazing TMJ and airway dentists, as well as a naturopath that introduced her to the dental meridian chart .

Linda's passionate goal in life is to help 1 million people who suffer from migraine headaches, TMJ, airway disorders, ADHD and fibromyalgia.

She is well on her way to reaching her goal.

**If you are interested in having Linda
do a presentation on fibromyalgia
or give an interview about her book, contact her at
fibromyalgiasecret@gmail.com or 586-612-4999**